FROM
PATIENT TO PAYMENT

Insurance Procedures for the Medical Office

FOURTH EDITION

Cynthia Newby, CPC

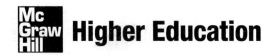 **Higher Education**

Boston   Burr Ridge, IL   Dubuque, IA   Madison, WI   New York   San Francisco   St. Louis
Bangkok   Bogotá   Caracas   Kuala Lumpur   Lisbon   London   Madrid   Mexico City
Milan   Montreal   New Delhi   Santiago   Seoul   Singapore   Sydney   Taipei   Toronto

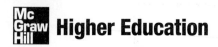

Higher Education

FROM PATIENT TO PAYMENT: INSURANCE PROCEDURES FOR THE MEDICAL OFFICE
FOURTH EDITION

Published by McGraw-Hill, a business unit of The McGraw-Hill Companies, Inc., 1221 Avenue of the Americas, New York, NY 10020. Copyright ©2005, 2002, 1998, 1993 by The McGraw-Hill Companies, Inc. All rights reserved. No part of this publication may be reproduced or distributed in any form or by any means, or stored in a database or retrieval system, without the prior written consent of The McGraw-Hill Companies, Inc., including, but not limited to, in any network or other electronic storage or transmission, or broadcast for distance learning.

Some ancillaries, including electronic and print components, may not be available to customers outside the United States.

 This book is printed on recycled, acid-free paper containing 10% postconsumer waste.

1 2 3 4 5 6 7 8 9 0 QPD/QPD 0 9 8 7 6 5 4

ISBN 0–07–301467–2

Publisher: *David T. Culverwell*
Senior Sponsoring Editor: *Roxan Kinsey*
Developmental Editor: *Patricia Forrest*
Editorial Coordinator: *Connie Kuhl*
Senior Marketing Manager: *James F. Connely*
Project Manager: *Cindy Schmerbach*
Production Supervisor: *Kara Kudronowicz*
Senior Media Project Manager: *Sandra M. Schnee*
Media Technology Producer: *Janna Martin*
Designer: *Laurie B. Janssen*
Cover Designer: *Studio Montage*
(USE) Cover Image: *Elite Images*
Supplement Producer: *Brenda A. Ernzen*
Compositor: *Lithokraft*
Typeface: *11.5/13 Minion*
Printer: *Quebecor World Dubuque, IA*

All brand or product names are trademarks or registered trademarks of their respective companies.

CPT five-digit codes, nomenclature, and other data are copyright ©2003 American Medical Association. All Rights Reserved. No fee schedules, basic units relative values, or related listings are included in CPT. The AMA assumes no liability for the data contained herein.

CPT codes are based on CPT 2004.
ICD-9-CM codes are based on ICD-9-CM 2004.

The Student Data Disk, illustrations, instructions, and exercises in *From Patient to Payment: Insurance Procedures for the Medical Office, Fourth Edition,* are compatible with the MediSoft Patient Accounting for Windows software available at the time of publication. Adaptations may be necessary for use with subsequent versions of the software. Text changes will be made in reprints when possible.

All names, situations, and anecdotes are fictitious. They do not represent any person, event, or medical record.

www.mhhe.com

Brief Contents

Contents

Preface

This text/workbook is designed for introductory medical insurance courses. Its practical, focused approach provides students with the basics of preparing correct health care claims.

Chapter Structure

Each chapter begins with four sections that provide a preview of what the student will study:

- *Objectives*—Describes the basic knowledge that can be acquired by studying the chapter.
- *Key Terms*—Presents an alphabetic list of important vocabulary terms found in the chapter. Key terms are printed in color type and defined when introduced in the text.
- *Why This Chapter Is Important to You*—Explains how the information in the chapter relates to the job of a medical insurance specialist.
- *What Do You Think?*—Describes a situation or discussion point for the student to consider.

The body of each chapter provides essential background information and practical, up-to-date procedures. Many figures and tables are included to enhance the learning process.

A *Chapter Summary* at the end of each chapter is followed by *Check Your Understanding*, which tests the student's knowledge of the chapter's key terms and content. Case studies, which test the application of the chapter's materials, appear either in the body of the chapter or in the *Check Your Understanding* section.

Special Features

Various feature boxes are included throughout the text:

- *HIPPA Tip*—Information for applying HIPAA privacy, security, and correct code sets in medical offices.
- *Professional Focus*—Facts about current computer technology, legislation, changing regulations, and career applications.
- *FYI*—"For Your Information" boxes with interesting bits of information about topics in the main text.
- *Compliance Tip*—Hints on the best ways to complete health care claims and on correctly handling situations that may arise in the medical office.
- *Explore the Internet*—Information about useful Web sites.

NDCMediSoft Claim Simulations

Because of the increasing importance of information technology in medical billing, Chapter 16 contains:

- Instructions for using the MediSoft medical billing program database located on the Student Data Disk
- Examples of claim preparation using MediSoft
- Five case studies to test the student's ability to process various types of insurance claims using MediSoft.

NDCMediSoft is free to adopters of *From Patient to Payment,* Fourth Edition; information on ordering and installing the software is located in the *Instructor's Manual* that accompanies the text. The Student Data Disk that comes with the text provides a base of case study information to be used with these computerized simulations.

The following equipment and supplies are needed for the computer simulations in Chapter 16:

- IBM or IBM-compatible computer with Pentium III or faster processor, 64 MB RAM, and 1 gig hard drive (500 MB available hard drive space)
- Microsoft Windows 98 (with current updates), Windows Me, Windows NT (Version 4 with current updates), Windows 2000, or Windows XP operating system
- NDCMediSoft Advanced, Version 9 *(free to adopters)*
- *From Patient to Payment* Student Data Disk
- A blank, formatted 3.5 floppy diskette
- Mouse or compatible pointing device
- CD-ROM 2X or faster
- Printer

Instructor's Manual for *From Patient to Payment,* Fourth Edition

The Instructor's Manual provides answers to the case studies and *Check Your Understanding* questions in the text, teaching suggestions, resources for insurance information, correlation charts for SCANS, the National Health Care Skill Standards, the 1997 AAMA Role Delineation Study Areas of Competence, and the AMT competencies. It also includes information on ordering and installing NDCMediSoft Patient Accounting software for Windows. The CD-ROM packaged with the Instructor's Manual includes PowerPoint Presentations highlighting the main points of each chapter and ExamView® Pro Test Generator.

Additional Medical Coding Materials

Since medical insurance specialists verify diagnosis and procedure codes and use them to report physicians' services, a fundamental understanding of coding principles and guidelines is the baseline for correct claims. Two options for additional coding experience are available.

1. For students with considerable training in medical coding, the *Medical Insurance Coding Workbook for Physician Practices* provides practice and instruction in coding and compliance skills. The workbook

reinforces and enhances skill development by applying basic coding principles and extending knowledge through additional coding guidelines, examples, and compliance tips. The workbook, which is updated each year, is also accompanied by an Instructor's Manual.

2. For students with limited exposure to medical coding, such as that provided by studying *From Patient to Payment,* Fourth Edition, the instructor may choose to assign **Basic Medical Coding For Physician Practices.** This text/workbook combines additional instruction in medical coding principles with the exercises from the *Medical Insurance Coding Workbook* to offer a complete basic medical coding course.

Acknowledgments

A number of people made significant contributions to the fourth edition of *From Patient to Payment.* For insightful reviews, criticisms, helpful suggestions, and information, we would like to acknowledge the following:

Emil Asdurian, M.D.
Drake Business School-Medical Program

Marion I. Bucci
Delaware Technical and Community College

Susan Dengler
Prince Georges Community College

Marilyn Graham
Moore Norman Technology Center

Richard Holley
Globe Institute of Technology; National Health Career Association

Elizabeth Keene, BSN, RN
Lansdale School of Business

Terri M. Kilpatrick NHE, LPN, RT ®, ROT, CPT
Apollo College, Albuquerque, NM

Melinda L. Loyst
Academy of Healing Arts

Patricia F. Rodgers
DuBois Business College (PA)
Huntington County Campus

Deborah Warner
DuBois Business College (PA)

Danny L. Webb (AMT), A+, A.S.
Golden State University

Kathy F. Wood, FHFMA
Catawba Valley Community College

To the Student

Welcome to *From Patient to Payment*. The NDCMedisoft software that you will use in Chapter 16: NDCMedisoft Claim Simulations will already be installed for your use. The data file that you will use with NDCMedisoft is provided on the Student Data Disk, which is included in two formats: floppy disk and CD-ROM. Detailed instructions for restoring the file from either format are provided in Chapter 16. Here are those instructions in brief:

1. Hold down the F7 key and start NDCMedisoft. When the Find NDCMedisoft Database dialog box appears, release the F7 key. Enter *C:\MediData* (where C is the letter that represents the hard drive you will be using) and click OK.
2. When the message, "This is not an existing root data directory. Do you want to create a new one?" appears, click Yes.
3. Click the Create a New Set of Data button. In the upper box, enter *Central Practice Center.* In the lower box, key *CPC.* Click the Create button.
4. When the Confirm dialog box is displayed, click Yes.
5. In the Practice Name box, key *Central Practice Center.* Click the Save button. The main window of the NDCMedisoft program is displayed.
6. Insert the Student Data Disk in the appropriate drive (floppy or CD-ROM).
7. Select Restore Data on the File menu. When the Warning dialog box is displayed, click OK.
8. In the top box of the Restore dialog box, key *X:\CPC.mbk,* where X is the letter of the drive that contains the Student Data Disk. Click the Start Restore button.
9. When the Confirm dialog box is displayed, click OK.
10. After the database is restored, a message appears, indicating that the restore is complete. Click OK.
11. When the main NDCMedisoft window reappears, select Open Practice on the File menu.
12. Central Practice Center is highlighted. To open the database file, click the OK button. You are returned to the main NDCMedisoft window. (*Hint:* If the main NDCMedisoft window does not fill the screen, click the Maximize button to expand it.)
13. By default, NDCMedisoft displays a sidebar with four options on the left side of the window. As the sidebar is not required for this text, open the Window menu and click the Show Side Bar option to toggle it off. The database is now ready for use.

CHAPTER 1

From Patient to Payment

Objectives

After completing this chapter, you will be able to define the key terms and:

1. Explain the main differences between indemnity plans and managed care plans.
2. Define the various types of insurance coverage.
3. Identify five steps in the health care claim billing and payment cycle.
4. List four primary responsibilities of a medical insurance specialist.
5. Discuss effects of health care claim errors on medical office routines.

Key Terms

assignment of benefits
benefits
coinsurance
copayment
deductible
dependent
diagnosis
direct payment
electronic claims
encounter form
fee-for-service
health care claim

health plan
indemnity plan
indirect payment
insurance carrier
managed care
managed care organization
    (MCO)
medical insurance
medical insurance specialist
patient information form
payer
policyholder

preauthorization
preexisting condition
premium
provider
remittance advice (RA)
schedule of benefits

Why This Chapter Is Important to You

The information in this chapter will enable you to:
- Understand the health care claim billing and payment cycle.
- Understand the role of a medical insurance specialist in a medical office.
- Understand the importance of working efficiently and accurately in a medical office.
- Begin to gain the skills that will make you a valuable member of a medical office staff.

What Do You Think?

The health care field is constantly changing. Costs for medical care are rising, and so is the demand for medical services. The majority of physicians are part of large group practices or clinics, rather than practicing alone. Patients have many choices in health care coverage and must select from a wide range of medical insurance options and prices. Thus, today's medical office staff often communicates with many insurance companies that have many different rules and policies regarding insurance claims. In what ways can the medical insurance specialist keep up-to-date concerning these issues?

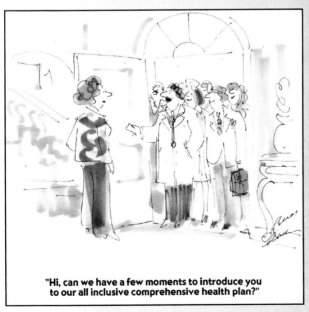

"Hi, can we have a few moments to introduce you to our all inclusive comprehensive health plan?"

Everyone, no matter how healthy, needs medical care at some time. People need preventive care, such as routine checkups and vaccinations, to stay healthy. They also need treatment for sicknesses, accidents, and injuries. A person who receives medical care owes a fee for the medical services involved. To be able to afford the charges, many people in the United States have medical insurance. Medical insurance is an agreement between a person, who is called the policyholder, and a health plan. Health plans, also known as insurance carriers or payers, are organizations that offer financial protection in case of illness or accidental injury. Medical insurance helps pay for the policyholder's medical treatment.

People buying medical insurance pay a premium to a health plan. In exchange for the premium, the health plan agrees to pay amounts, called benefits, for medical services. Medical services include the care supplied by providers—hospitals, physicians, and other medical staff and facilities.

The insurance policy contains a schedule of benefits, which is a list of covered medical services. Benefits commonly include payment of medically necessary medical treatments received by policyholders and their dependents. Typical medical services include surgery, primary care, emergency care, and specialists' services. Other medically related expenses, such as hospital-based services, are usually included. However, if a new policyholder has a medical condition that was diagnosed before the policy was written—known as a preexisting condition—a health plan may not cover medical services for the treatment of that condition.

Many health plans also cover preventive medical services, such as annual physical examinations, pediatric and adolescent immunizations, prenatal care, and routine cancer screening procedures such as mammograms. Policies also list treatments that are covered at different rates and noncovered services. For example, a plan may pay 80 percent of most physically related treatments but a smaller percentage of the charges for mental health services. Coverage for dental care is generally not included. However, separate dental insurance plans are available for purchase.

Indemnity Plans

In the last century, most medical insurance policies in the United States were indemnity plans. Under an indemnity plan, the medical costs policyholders incur when they receive treatment for accidents and illnesses are paid by the insurance carrier. If a policyholder or a covered dependent (a spouse, child, or other relative specified in the insurance policy) gets sick, the health plan pays most of the bill. Benefits are determined on a fee-for-service basis. In other words, benefits are based on the fees physicians charge for the services.

Under an indemnity plan, the policy lists the services that are paid for and the amounts that are paid. The benefit may be for all or part of the charges. In many cases, the policyholder owes a percentage of the fees, usually called coinsurance. For example, the schedule of benefits in a medical insurance policy may say it pays 80 percent of the fees for surgery performed in a hospital, and the policyholder must pay 20 percent. Under this contract, if the policyholder has surgery in the hospital and the bill is $2,000, the health plan pays 80 percent of $2,000, or $1,600. The policyholder is responsible for the coinsurance—the other 20 percent, or $400 in this example.

Managed Care Plans

Under indemnity plans, it is difficult for insurance carriers to control costs, because there have been few restrictions on providers' charges, especially for new technology, drugs, and procedures. To counter this trend, the concept of managed care has been introduced. Managed care is a way of supervising medical care with the goal of ensuring that patients get needed services in the most appropriate, cost-effective setting.

To accomplish managed care goals, the financing and management of health care are combined with the delivery of services. Managed care organizations (MCOs) establish links among provider, patient, and payer. Instead of only the patient's having a policy with the health plan, under managed care both the patient and the provider have agreements with the MCO. The patient agrees to the payments for the services, and the provider agrees to accept the fees the MCO offers for services. This arrangement gives the managed care plan more control over what services the provider performs and the fees the plan pays.

Managed care is the leading type of health plan, and many different kinds of managed care programs are available. These are covered in detail in Chapter 5. In some cases, patients pay fixed premiums at regular time periods, such as monthly. A patient may also pay a copayment—a small fixed fee, such as $10, for each office visit. In some plans, this "copay" is a percentage of the amount the provider receives. In either case, copayments must always be paid by the patient at the time of service.

Cost Containment

Most health plans, including indemnity plans, now have cost-containment practices to help control costs. For example, patients may be required to choose from a specific group of physicians and hospitals for all medical care. Visits to specialists often must be made by a referral from the patient's primary care physician. A second physician's opinion may be required before surgery can be reimbursed. Also, many services that previously involved overnight hospital stays are now covered only if done during daytime hospital visits, with patients recuperating at home.

Preauthorization is another example of a cost-containment practice. If preauthorization is required, the health plan must approve a procedure before it is done in order for the procedure to be covered. For example, many nonemergency services must be approved before a patient is admitted to the hospital. Also, shorter hospital stays are encouraged, and weekend hospital admissions for Monday services may not be permitted.

COMMON TYPES OF MEDICAL INSURANCE

Some patients seen in a medical office are covered by private insurance. Others qualify for programs sponsored by state or federal governments.

Private Insurance

Private health plans offer a variety of types of medical insurance coverage. Most are group contracts—policies that cover people who work for the same employer or belong to the same organization. Examples include private companies, professional associations, labor unions, and schools. Other plans are offered as individual contracts, which are policies purchased by people who do not qualify as members of a group.

Some employers have established themselves as self-insured health plans. Rather than paying a premium to an insurance carrier, the organization "insures itself." It assumes the risk of paying directly for medical services, establishes contracts with local physician practices, and sets up a fund with which it pays for claims. The organization itself establishes the benefit levels and the plan types it will offer.

People may also have medical coverage through their liability insurance and automotive insurance. For example, people injured in automobile accidents may be insured through the medical benefit of their or another party's automotive policy. Coverage varies by state.

Government Plans

The most common government plans in effect in the United States are:

- *Medicare*—Medicare is a federal health plan that covers citizens aged 65 (must have paid into FICA for at least 10 years) and over, people with disabilities, ESRD (certain transplants, such as kidney, and heart-lung), and dependent widows.
- *Medicaid*—Low-income people who cannot afford medical care are covered by Medicaid, which is cosponsored by federal and state governments. (Medicaid is a state-run program; there are matching federal dollars available for states that satisfy certain requirements, such as providing prenatal care and child vaccinations.) Qualifications and benefits vary by state.
- *Workers' Compensation*—People with job-related illnesses or injuries are covered under workers' compensation insurance through their employer. Workers' compensation benefits vary according to state law.
- *TRICARE (formerly CHAMPUS)*—This program covers expenses for dependents of active duty members of the uniformed services and for retired military personnel. It also covers dependents of military personnel who were killed while on active duty.
- *CHAMPVA*—The Civilian Health and Medical Program of the Department of Veterans Affairs is for veterans with permanent service-related disabilities and their dependents. It also covers surviving spouses and dependent children of veterans who died from service-related disabilities.

In most cases, a person covered by a health plan receives insurance benefits by filing a health care claim. This claim identifies the policyholder (and the patient, if this person is not the policyholder) and tells the health plan which medical services were performed and why. Most medical offices handle claim filing for patients, and processing health care claims is the responsibility of a medical insurance specialist.

There are five steps in the payment process of a patient's health care claim, as discussed below:

Step 1 The patient completes (or updates) the patient information form; insurance coverage is verified.

Step 2 The physician examines the patient, evaluates the patient's condition, treats the patient, and completes the patient's encounter form.

Step 3 The medical insurance specialist completes the health care claim and transmits it to the health plan.

Step 4 The health plan processes the claim, makes appropriate payment, and provides a remittance advice that explains how the payment was determined.

Step 5 The medical insurance specialist records payment, reviews the accompanying remittance advice for accuracy, and determines whether any additional payment is due from another insurance plan or from the patient.

Step 1 The patient completes (or updates) the patient information form.

A new patient who comes to a medical office usually fills out a patient information form, also known as a registration form. Returning patients are asked to check and update their patient information forms. Most medical offices make sure that patients' forms are updated at least every twelve months. As shown in Figure 1-1 on page 8, the patient information form provides the personal, employment, and medical insurance information needed to file a claim.

If the patient has insurance coverage, the medical office staff verifies coverage by communicating with the health plan to check that the patient will be covered for services being provided, and to find out the terms and conditions of the insurance coverage, such as whether a co-payment is required.

Patient information forms usually ask for the patient's signature or for a parent's or guardian's signature if the patient is a minor. As part of the form or separately, patients usually sign an assignment of benefits. The assignment of benefits is a statement that tells the health plan to pay benefits directly to the physician. If the patient does not sign the assignment of benefits, the insurance benefit check goes to the policyholder, who must then pay the provider. Another signature permits the provider to give the health plan information needed to help process the claim. Although providers have a right to do this under federal law without a patient's signature (explained in Chapter 2), most medical offices have patients also sign this line.

CENTRAL PRACTICE CENTER
1122 E. University Drive
Mesa, AZ 85204
602–969–4237

Patient				
Last Name	First Name	MI	Sex __ M __ F	Date of Birth / /
Address	City		State	Zip
Home Ph # ( )	Marital Status		Student Status	
SS#	Allergies:			
Employment Status	Employer Name	Work Ph # ( )	Primary Insurance ID#	
Employer Address	City		State	Zip
Referred By		Ph # of Referral ( )		

Responsible Party (Complete this section if the person responsible for the bill is not the patient)

Last Name	First Name	MI	Sex __ M __ F	Date of Birth / /
Address	City	State	Zip	SS#
Relation to Patient __ Spouse __ Parent __ Other	Employer Name		Work Phone # ( )	
Spouse, or Parent (if minor):			Home Phone # ( )	

Insurance (If you have multiple coverage, supply information from both carriers)

Primary Carrier Name	Secondary Carrier Name
Name of the Insured (Name on ID Card)	Name of the Insured (Name on ID Card)
Patient's relationship to the insured __ Self __ Spouse __ Child __ Other	Patient's relationship to the insured __ Self __ Spouse __ Child __ Other
Insured ID #	Insured ID #
Group # or Company Name	Group # or Company Name
Insurance Address	Insurance Address
Phone #	Copay $	Phone #	Copay $

Other Information

Is patient's condition related to:
__ Employment   __ Auto Accident (if yes, state in which accident occurred: ___)   __ Other Accident

Reason for visit: _____

Date of Accident: /   /   Date of First Symptom of Illness: /   /

Authorization

I hereby authorize release of information necessary for my insurance company to process my claim. The above information is correct to the best of my knowledge. Signed: _____Date: _____	I hereby authorize payment directly to CENTRAL PRACTICE CENTER insurance benefits otherwise payable to me. I understand that I am financially responsible for charges not paid in a timely manner by my insurance. Signed: _____Date: _____

Figure 1-1 Patient Information Form

The medical insurance specialist files the patient information form in the financial section of the patient's medical record. Patients' financial records include insurance and billing information. The patient's medical record is a file that also includes the patient's medical history, record of treatment and progress, and other communications.

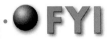
Step 2 The physician examines the patient, evaluates the patient's condition, treats the patient, and completes the patient's encounter form.

When the patient sees the physician, the complaint and symptom(s) are documented in the patient's medical record. Also listed are the diagnosis— the physician's opinion of the nature of the patient's illness or injury—and a description of tests and treatment, including any medicines prescribed.

The physician then fills out some type of encounter form. This form has space for the diagnosis, medical services, and fees for the day's visit. An example is shown in Figure 1-2 on page 10. Although the encounter form may be as simple as a receipt, usually it is a specially designed form. In some offices, it may be called a superbill or charge ticket. Encounter forms list procedures typical to a particular medical office.

Step 3 The medical insurance specialist completes the health care claim and transmits it to the health plan.

In most cases, the patient's encounter will be reported to the health plan using a standardized claim. (This claim is described in detail in Chapter 6.) Using information from the patient information form, the patient's medical record, and the patient's encounter form, the medical insurance specialist completes the health care claim.

Medical billing programs are typically used to prepare health care claims. Billing programs streamline the important process of creating and following up on claims sent to health plans and bills sent to patients.

The claim requires coding that uses letters and numbers to identify the diagnosis and procedures. Either the medical insurance specialist or a medical coder looks up the proper codes for the patient's diagnosis and procedures and records them on the insurance claim.

The completed claim is recorded in the billing program's insurance log, a running list of insurance claims that have been sent to all carriers. The health care claim is then sent to the health plan in one of two ways. Most claims are electronic claims sent by transferring information from a computer in the provider's office to a health plan's computer. The other type, paper claims, are printed and mailed to the payer.

Step 4 The health plan processes the claim, makes appropriate payment, and provides a remittance advice that explains how the payment was determined.

At the health plan's office, the claim is processed by the claims department. The diagnosis and procedures are reviewed to be sure the treatment was medically necessary, which means appropriate for the diagnosis.

To use an extreme example, suppose the codes on the claim indicate that the patient had a broken arm and that the procedure was removal of the tonsils. Since removing the tonsils is not a medically necessary treatment for a broken arm, the claim would be denied. If the patient was treated with a cast for the broken arm instead, it would suit the diagnosis and would be considered medically necessary.

CENTRAL PRACTICE CENTER

1122 E. University Drive
Mesa, AZ 85204
602–969–4237

PATIENT NAME				APPT. DATE/TIME			

PATIENT NO.				DX			
				1.			
				2.			
				3.			
				4.			

DESCRIPTION	✓	CPT	FEE	DESCRIPTION	✓	CPT	FEE
EXAMINATION				**PROCEDURES**			
New Patient				Diagnostic Anoscopy		46600	
Problem Focused		99201		ECG Complete		93000	
Expanded Problem Focused		99202		I&D, Abscess		10060	
Detailed		99203		Pap Smear		88150	
Comprehensive		99204		Removal of Cerumen		69210	
Comprehensive/Complex		99205		Removal 1 Lesion		17000	
Established Patient				Removal 2-14 Lesions		17003	
Minimum		99211		Removal 15+ Lesions		17004	
Problem Focused		99212		Rhythm ECG w/Report		93040	
Expanded Problem Focused		99213		Rhythm ECG w/Tracing		93041	
Detailed		99214		Sigmoidoscopy, diag.		45330	
Comprehensive/Complex		99215					
				LABORATORY			
PREVENTIVE VISIT				Bacteria Culture		87081	
New Patient				Fungal Culture		87101	
Age 12-17		99384		Glucose Finger Stick		82948	
Age 18-39		99385		Lipid Panel		80061	
Age 40-64		99386		Specimen Handling		99000	
Age 65+		99387		Stool/Occult Blood		82270	
Established Patient				Tine Test		85008	
Age 12-17		99394		Tuberculin PPD		85590	
Age 18-39		99395		Urinalysis		81000	
Age 40-64		99396		Venipuncture		36415	
Age 65+		99397					
				INJECTION/IMMUN.			
CONSULTATION: OFFICE/ER				DT Immun		90702	
Requested By:				Hepatitis A Immun		90632	
Problem Focused		99241		Hepatitis B Immun		90746	
Expanded Problem Focused		99242		Influenza Immun		90659	
Detailed		99243		Pneumovax		90732	
Comprehensive		99244					
Comprehensive/Complex		99245					
				TOTAL FEES			

Figure 1-2 Encounter form

The claims department compares the services to the schedule of benefits in the patient's policy and determines the amount of benefit to be paid on the claim. Many plans include a deductible, an amount of money the policyholder must pay before insurance benefits are paid. Only medical services that are covered in the schedule of benefits count toward the deductible.

For example, suppose Glenda Williams's plan has a $250 annual deductible. This means that her insurance company does not pay any benefits until she has spent $250 for services covered by her policy. If her medical bills total $400, she must pay the first $250. The insurance carrier will pay part or all of the remaining $150 according to the schedule of benefits in her policy.

Once the amount of benefit is determined, the insurance company issues a check. At the same time, it issues a remittance advice (RA). As shown in Figure 1-3, this document shows how the amount of benefit was determined. The insurance carrier may send payment to the physician or to the policyholder. If payment goes directly to the physician, it is called a direct payment. If it goes to the policyholder, it is an indirect payment. In either case, the patient receives a document that explains the payment, as shown in Figure 1-4 on page 12. Note that the RA is often also called an explanation of benefits (EOB).

Anthem Blue Cross Blue Shield
900 West Market Street
Phoenix, AZ 84209
Date prepared: 6/22/2008

Patient's name	Dates of service from - thru	POS	Proc	Qty	Charge amount	Eligible amount	Patient liability	Amt paid provider
Claim number 0347914								
Daiute, Angelo X	06/17/08 - 06/17/08	11	36415	1	$11.00	$11.00	$00.00	$11.00
Daiute, Angelo X	06/17/08 - 06/17/08	11	80050	1	$98.00	$98.00	$00.00	$98.00
Daiute, Angelo X	06/17/08 - 06/17/08	11	81000	1	$12.00	$12.00	$00.00	$12.00
Daiute, Angelo X	06/17/08 - 06/17/08	11	93000	1	$51.00	$51.00	$00.00	$51.00
Daiute, Angelo X	06/17/08 - 06/17/08	11	99386	1	$123.00	$123.00	$00.00	$123.00

Figure 1-3 Sample Remittance Advice

Step 5 The medical insurance specialist records payment, reviews the accompanying benefits explanation for accuracy, and determines whether additional payment is due from the patient.

When the RA arrives at the physician's office, the medical insurance specialist reviews it, checks all calculations, and makes sure that all charges submitted were processed and that the amounts paid are correct. If an error is found, a request for a review of the claim must be filed with the carrier.

The specialist next records the payment information in the medical billing program. If the patient has more than one insurance plan, the cycle is repeated, and the claim and payment information is sent to the second payer. The billing program is used to determine whether the patient owes any additional payment on the account. If so, the staff bills the remaining balance to the patient. An example of a bill sent to a patient is shown in Figure 1-5 on page 13.

CUSTOMER'S EXPLANATION OF BENEFITS

THIS IS NOT A BILL. RETAIN FOR YOUR RECORDS.

1324 0664402

CUSTOMER'S NAME: SUSAN BILTON
ID NUMBER: 140385526
PATIENT'S NAME: SUSAN BILTON

COVERAGE: BCBS OF NJ

CONSUMER DIVISION

CLAIM NUMBER: 7970920006160000
CLAIM RECEIVED: 04/02/2004
CLAIM FINALIZED: 04/08/2004
CHECK NUMBER: 0005890315

MEDICAL SURGICAL/MAJOR MEDICAL CLAIM SUMMARY

CHARGES FOR THIS CLAIM..$ 1,224.00
AMOUNT OF CUSTOMER BALANCE REMAINING ....$ 367.20
BENEFITS PAID TO SUSAN BILTON ....$ 856.80

DO NOT SUBMIT A SEPARATE MAJOR MEDICAL CLAIM FORM
THIS CLAIM HAS BEEN PROCESSED UNDER YOUR MEDICAL-SURGICAL AND MAJOR MEDICAL CONTRACTS

PATIENT'S NAME: SUSAN BILTON **IDENTIFICATION NUMBER: 140385526** **CLAIM NUMBER: 7970920006160000**

PROVIDER NAME / TYPE OF SERVICE - PLACE OF SERVICE	DATE OF SERVICE FROM TO	1 CHARGE AMOUNT	2 OTHER INS PAYMENT	3 NOT COVERED AMOUNT	4 ELIGIBLE AMOUNT	5 DEDUC-TIBLE	6 COINS/ CO-PAY	7 BENEFIT AMOUNT	8 CUSTOMER BALANCE	9 MSG CODES
ANESTHESIA CONSLTNTS CENTRL JERSEY										
ANESTHESIA-INPATIENT	03/13/04 03/13/04	1224.00			1224.00		367.20	856.80		
MAJOR MEDICAL		1224.00						0.00	367.20	
TOTALS		1224.00			1224.00		367.20	856.80	367.20	

THIS IS NOT A BILL

MESSAGES

CRP02B (1-97)

* SUSAN HAS SATISFIED $1,000.00 OF HER DEDUCTIBLE FOR THE PERIOD 01-01-04 TO 12-31-04. (0055)

Figure 1-4 Sample Patient Explanation of Benefits

Explore the Internet

Using the search engine of your choosing, explore the job statistics gathered by the Bureau of Labor Statistics. At the Bureau's home page, choose Keyword Search of BLS Web Pages, and enter a job title of interest to you. Two suggested choices for your search are (1) medical assistants and (2) health information technicians. In particular, review the job outlook information.

CENTRAL PRACTICE CENTER
1122 E. University Drive
Mesa, AZ 85204

Statement Date	Page
10/13/2008	1

Vereen Williams
17 Mill Rd
Chandler, AZ 85246-4567

Chart Number
WILLIVE0

Date	Document	Description	Case Number	Amount
			Previous Balance:	0.00

Patient: Walter Williams — Chart # WILLIWA0
Case Description: Hypertension — Last Payment Received: 10/1/2008 — Amount: -15.00

Date	Document	Description	Case Number	Amount
10/1/2008	0810010000	EP Problem Focused	8	46.00
10/1/2008	0810010000	ECG Complete	8	70.00
10/1/2008	0810010000	Aetna Copayment Charge	8	15.00
10/1/2008	0810010000	Aetna Copayment	8	-15.00

Past Due 30 Days	Past Due 60 Days	Past Due 90 Days	Balance Due
0.00	0.00	0.00	**116.00**

Figure 1-5 Sample Patient Invoice

Professional Focus

The Internet and Medical Insurance

The World Wide Web is a valuable source of information about many topics of interest to medical insurance specialists. For example, many insurance carriers have Web sites that post updates to their claims submission procedures. Professional organizations, such as the American Medical Association, offer information and opinions on timely medical topics.

Each chapter of this text contains an Explore the Internet box that suggests a Web site that may be of use to you. Visit these sites and begin to build a reference library of resources that will help you in your future role as a medical insurance specialist.

THE RESPONSIBILITIES OF A MEDICAL INSURANCE SPECIALIST

The medical insurance specialist plays an important role in the daily business routine of a medical office. A key responsibility is smoothing the way for payments from health plans and from patients. The work includes much more than filling in blanks on a health care claim. It requires knowledge of the insurance process and the ability to work with a variety of complex insurance plans.

Physicians and, often, the practice manager determine the medical insurance specialist's job duties. Although parts of the job may vary, most medical insurance specialists perform similar tasks. Examples include gathering patient information and signatures, filing health care claims, reviewing payments, and helping patients understand insurance procedures.

The following are some duties involved in these responsibilities:

Gather and Verify Information

- Obtain and update information on patient information forms, and file forms in patients' medical records.
- Verify patients' insurance coverage, and secure any needed preauthorizations.
- Ask patients for appropriate signatures authorizing assignment of benefits.
- Find diagnoses, treatments, and charges on the encounter forms in patients' medical records.

Use a Medical Billing Program to Prepare and Submit Health Care Claims

- Enter accurate patient information, such as names, addresses, and birth dates.
- Verify insurance carriers' names and addresses.
- Enter complete and accurate information for the patient's visit, including correct codes for all diagnoses and procedures.
- Check the charges for each service, and enter any payment the patient made toward the claim, if applicable.
- Submit claims by electronic transmission or mail.

Review Insurance Payments

- Follow up on claims to ensure prompt payment.
- Review remittance advices, checking for errors in calculations. Be sure all submitted charges have been considered by the payer.
- Request reviews by health plans when reimbursement appears to be in error.
- Enter payments that are received in patients' accounts, and bill any balances due, if appropriate.
- Coordinate with the physicians and practice manager to answer payers' requests for more information.

Help Patients

- Answer patients' questions about insurance reimbursement and the health care claim process.
- Assist patients when problems with payers arise.

EFFECTS OF HEALTH CARE CLAIM ERRORS

Efficient and accurate completion of the health care claim process helps a medical office run smoothly. The job of the medical insurance specialist is important, because most of the income received in a medical office comes from insurance payments. Errors in filing claims slow the reimbursement process and interfere with other work. Some examples of problems that can arise from filing inaccurate claims include the following:

Lower Payments and Denied Claims

A typographical error or incorrect code will give the payer the wrong diagnosis or treatment. This can result in a lower benefit payment or denial of the claim.

Delays in Payments

If the health plan must request additional information, payment will be delayed. The payer's claims department can correct an error, but it takes time, so issuing the benefit payment will take longer.

Disruption of Other Work

When a medical insurance specialist has to correct a claim form or fill out a request for a review, the time spent means that new claims for other patients have to wait. Correcting information may also require the assistance of the physician or other members of the office staff, who then must interrupt their activities.

Patients' Questions and Complaints

If a patient has already paid for services, errors in the claim process can slow reimbursement. The medical insurance specialist or another member of the office staff may have to interrupt activities to handle inquiries and complaints.

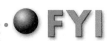

Some services performed by physicians do not take place in medical offices but rather in other locations, such as hospitals. When a patient is admitted to a hospital, the medical insurance specialist is responsible for gathering complete and correct information. Hospitals may send reports to the physician's office. These reports are used to complete health care forms.

1. Health plans pay for patients' medical services according to the policy's schedule of benefits. Most health plans require premiums to be paid. Some plans pay a percentage of the charge, while others require just a copayment. Under managed care plans, which are the most popular plans, providers' fees are set in advance. Most health plans now have some cost-containment features.

2. Common kinds of private medical insurance include group insurance, individual insurance, liability insurance, and automotive insurance. Government programs include Medicare, Medicaid, workers' compensation, TRICARE, and CHAMPVA.

3. The five steps in the health care billing and payment process are:

   (a) The patient completes (or updates) the patient information form; insurance coverage is verified.

   (b) The physician examines the patient, evaluates the patient's condition, treats the patient, and completes the patient's encounter form.

   (c) The medical insurance specialist completes the health care claim and transmits it to the health plan.

   (d) The health plan processes the claim, makes appropriate payment, and provides a remittance advice that explains how the payment was determined.

   (e) The medical insurance specialist records payment, reviews the accompanying remittance advice for accuracy, and determines whether additional payment is due from another insurance plan or from the patient.

4. The four main duties performed by the medical insurance specialist are:

   (a) Gather and verify information.

   (b) Use a medical billing program to prepare and submit health care claims.

   (c) Review insurance payments, post payments, and follow up billing.

   (d) Help patients.

5. Insurance claim errors slow the reimbursement process and interfere with other work in the medical office. Effects of errors include lower payments and denied claims, delays in payments, disruption of other work, and increased questions and complaints by patients.

Check Your Understanding

Part 1. Put the five steps in the billing and payment process in the correct order.

    a. Physician examines the patient, evaluates the patient's condition, treats the patient, and completes the patient's encounter form.

    b. Patient completes (or updates) the patient information form.

    c. Health plan processes the claim, makes appropriate payment, and provides a remittance advice.

    d. Medical insurance specialist records payment, reviews the accompanying remittance advice for accuracy, and determines whether the patient owes any additional payment.

    e. Medical insurance specialist completes the health care claim and transmits it to the health plan.

Part 2. Choose the best answer.

_____ **1.** The amount an insurance carrier will pay for a covered medical service is the
    a. benefit
    b. premium
    c. claim

_____ **2.** Under an indemnity plan, benefits are determined on what basis?
    a. fee-for-service
    b. cost-containment
    c. either a or b

_____ **3.** Under a managed care plan, fixed fees for medical procedures and services are set by the
    a. health care provider
    b. managed care organization
    c. patient

_____ **4.** The patient information form gives information about
    a. the patient
    b. the insurance company
    c. both a and b

_____ **5.** The file that contains the patient's medical and insurance information is the
    a. encounter form
    b. patient's medical record
    c. code

_____ **6.** The amount of money a patient must pay before the health plan will pay for services (list all that apply):
    a. benefit
    b. premium
    c. deductible

_____ **7.** The medical billing program is used to record
    a. claims sent
    b. health plans' payments
    c. both a and b

_____ **8.** When treatment is appropriate for the patient's diagnosis, it is said to be
    a. medically necessary
    b. deductible
    c. direct

_____ **9.** The assignment of benefits allows the health plan to
    a. pay the physician for services
    b. withhold payments for services
    c. pay the patient for services

_____ **10.** Coding means
    a. writing prescriptions so patients cannot read them
    b. assigning proper numbers to identify the diagnoses and procedures on claims
    c. using a billing program for the patient's progress notes

Part 3. Write "T" or "F" in the blank to indicate whether you think the statement is true or false.

_____ **1.** The job of the medical insurance specialist is not really very important in a medical office.

_____ **2.** The job description of a medical insurance specialist is determined by the physicians and practice manager.

_____ **3.** The encounter form lists the diagnosis, medical services, and fees for a patient's visit.

_____ **4.** The medical insurance specialist files the patient information form in the patient's medical record.

_____ **5.** The only duty a medical insurance specialist has is to transmit health care claims to insurance carriers.

_____ **6.** Finding the correct codes for diagnosis and treatment is performed by the medical specialist or a medical coder.

_____ **7.** Once the health care claim is transmitted to the payer, the job of the medical insurance specialist is finished.

_____ **8.** If a patient calls with a question about insurance, the call should be directed to the physician.

_____ **9.** The term _remittance advice_ means that the medical insurance specialist explains insurance problems to the patient.

_____ **10.** If there seems to be a mistake in the amount of money paid by an insurance carrier, the medical insurance specialist should request a review.

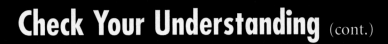

Part 4. Match the following insurance programs to the patients who qualify for them. Note that some letters are used more than one time.

A. TRICARE
B. CHAMPVA
C. Medicare
D. Medicaid
E. workers' compensation
F. individual insurance
G. group insurance

_____ **1.** Tom Kahler is seventy-three years old.

_____ **2.** Linda Belize hurt her back lifting a case of motor oil in the warehouse at work.

_____ **3.** Amy Jenks is the five-year-old daughter of a U.S. Army sergeant stationed in Korea.

_____ **4.** Rachel Marinaccio is a vice president of First Bank, where she participates in the company's health insurance plan.

_____ **5.** Cynthia Weiner's husband died of complications from paralysis that resulted from stepping on a land mine when he was a U.S. Marine during the Vietnam war.

_____ **6.** Jill Ludwig receives state welfare benefits.

_____ **7.** Captain Cheryl Kupper is retired from the U.S. Navy.

_____ **8.** Emelina Valdez subscribes to health insurance through the same agent who carries her automobile and homeowner's insurance.

_____ **9.** Kenji Ito has a permanent disability not related to service in the armed forces or a work-related injury.

_____**10.** Thurman Jackson is covered by his wife's insurance through the Automobile Dealers' Association.

2 HIPAA and the Legal Medical Record

Objectives

After completing this chapter, you will be able to define the key terms and:

1. Discuss the importance of medical record documentation in the billing and payment process.
2. Define the facts that are included in patients' protected health information (PHI).
3. Discuss the purpose of the HIPAA Privacy Rule.
4. Describe what PHI can be released without patients' authorization.
5. Discuss patients' authorizations to use or disclose PHI.
6. Describe the purpose of a retention schedule.
7. Discuss how to guard against potentially fraudulent situations.

Key Terms

Acknowledgment of Receipt
  of Notice of Privacy
  Practices
authorization
clearinghouse
compliance plan
documentation
fraud

Health Insurance Portability
  and Accountability Act
  (HIPAA)
HIPAA Privacy Rule
medical records
minimum necessary standard
Notice of Privacy Practices
Office of Civil Rights (OCR)

protected health information
  (PHI)
retention schedule
subpoena
subpoena *duces tecum*
treatment, payment,
  and operations (TPO)

Why This Chapter Is Important to You

The information in this chapter will enable you to:

- Understand the importance of keeping medical records private and secure.
- Feel confident about how to respond when someone requests information about a patient.
- Know how to protect yourself, the physician, and other staff members from potentially fraudulent situations.

What Do You Think?

The work of physicians involves many legal issues, such as possible accusations of false billing or of incorrectly disclosing a patient's private information. The work of the medical insurance specialist also involves many legal considerations. Not only must patients' protected health information be respected and kept confidential, but physicians must also be guarded from potentially fraudulent situations. For example, a patient may attempt to persuade the medical insurance specialist to change a fact on a claim in order to receive benefits falsely. In your opinion, is it ever appropriate for a medical insurance specialist to alter a claim?

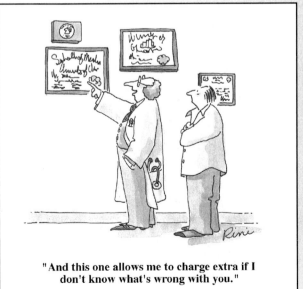

"And this one allows me to charge extra if I don't know what's wrong with you."

Patients' medical records contain all facts, findings, and observations about their health history. They also contain all communications with and about each patient. The medical record in the medical office begins with a patient's first contact and continues through all treatments and services. These records provide continuity and communication among physicians and other health care professionals who are involved in a patient's care. Patient medical records are also used in research and for education.

Patient medical records are legal documents. Physicians own the physical record (although patients "own" information about them), and properly documented patient care is part of a physician's defense against accusations that patients were not treated correctly. Medical records should clearly state who performed what service and describe why, where, when, and how it was done. Physicians document the rationale behind their treatment decisions. This rationale is the basis for the concept of medical necessity—a clinically logical link between a patient's condition and the treatment provided. For example, when a test or drug is ordered for a patient, the physician documents the diagnosis or condition that is being confirmed or ruled out.

Although they do not make entries in patient medical records, medical insurance specialists work with the records in the billing and payment process. The documentation of diagnoses and procedures is used as proof of billed services. An unwritten law of medical insurance is that if it was not documented, it was not done, and if it was not done, it cannot be billed. Payers also use documentation to decide whether the reported services should be reimbursed. The record must clearly document where, why, when, and how each service occurred.

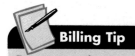

Billing Tip

Documentation and Billing

The connection between documentation and billing bears repeating: If a service is not documented, it was not done, and if it was not done, it cannot be billed.

Documentation Standards

In medical record documentation, a patient's health status is recorded in chronological order using a systematic, logical, and consistent method. A patient's health history, examinations, tests, and results of treatments are all documented. Because of the importance of patients' medical records, the leading health care industry groups set standards for documentation. Standardization helps make medical records more efficient and improves the quality of patient care. Since medical insurance specialists help organize and maintain patient medical records, it is important to be aware of these standards and encourage their use:

- *Records must be clear:* Medical records should be complete and accurate. If the records are handwritten, the entries should be legible to others, made in black ink (not pencil), and dated.

- *Entries must be signed and dated:* Whether digitally entered by the provider, handwritten, or transcribed, each entry must have the signature or initials and title of the responsible provider and the date.

- *Changes must be clearly made:* An incorrect entry is marked with a single line through the words to be changed; the correct information is entered after it, so that the previous copy can be read. Corrections are also dated and signed by the person making the change. No part of a record should be otherwise altered or removed, deleted, or destroyed.

Example

Correct	Incorrect	Guideline
85 5/7/2007 this ~~80~~-year old *jrb*	85 this ~~8~~-year old	Corrections should be clear, signed, and dated.

- *No blank spaces may be left between entries:* Entries are made chronologically, without spaces between them, to prevent out-of-order entries.
- *Each patient should have a single record:* Each patient should have one medical record, often called a unit record. (Note, however, that practices should be sure to have a separate file in a patient's medical record when workers' compensation claims are involved; see Chapter 12.)
- *Records should use consistent vocabulary and format:* All entries should reflect standard, accepted medical vocabulary and abbreviations. All medical records in a practice should be consistently labeled and have logical sections.
- *Diagnostic information must be easy to locate:* Past and present diagnoses should be placed so that they are easy to locate by each physician who uses the medical record.
- *Practitioners' entries must be made promptly:* Entries should be made in a timely manner and filed in a consistent chronological order, either ascending or descending.

Documentation Formats

Medical insurance specialists work with various formats that are used to organize patients' medical records. The most common format used in general medical practices is called a *problem-oriented medical record* (POMR). The problem-oriented medical record contains a general section with data from the initial patient examination and assessment. When the patient makes subsequent visits, the reasons for those encounters are listed separately in a problem list, each with its own notes. For example, the patient's record might have a general section followed by sections labeled "skin disorder" and "right eye scleral abrasion" with notes about these conditions.

Progress notes for each problem are in the SOAP format, beginning with the problem and then four points: *Subjective, Objective, Assessment,* and *Plan:*

S: The *subjective* information is based on the patient's descriptions of symptoms along with other comments.

O: The *objective* information includes the physical examinations and laboratory reports or tests.

A: The *assessment,* also called the impression or conclusion, is the physician's diagnosis, or interpretation of the subjective and objective information.

P: The *plan,* also called treatment, advice, or recommendations, includes the necessary patient monitoring, follow-up, procedures, and instructions to the patient.

Documentation Content

Providers follow generally recognized guidelines to document encounters. The initial examinations and assessments (see Figure 2-1) show the treatment plan for the patient. Progress reports document the patient's progress and response to the treatment plan (see Figure 2-2). Discharge summaries are prepared during the patient's final visit for a particular treatment plan. If either the patient or the physician ends the relationship, the physician must still maintain the patient's medical record. The physician also sends the patient a letter that documents the situation and provides for continuity of care with the next provider.

James E. Ribielli
5/19/2008

CHIEF COMPLAINT: This 79-year-old male presents with sudden and extreme weakness. He got up from a seated position and became light-headed.

PAST MEDICAL HISTORY: History of congestive heart failure. On multiple medications, including Cardizem, Enalapril 5 mg qd, and Lasix 40 mg qd.

PHYSICAL EXAMINATION: No postural change in blood pressure. BP, 114/61 with a pulse of 49, sitting; BP, 111/56 with a pulse 50, standing. Patient denies being light-headed at this time.

    HEENT: Unremarkable.

    NECK: Supple without jugular or venous distension.

    LUNGS: Clear to auscultation and percussion.

    HEART: S1 and S2 normal; no systolic or diastolic murmurs; no S3, S4. No dysrhythmia.

    ABDOMEN: Soft without organomegaly, mass, or bruit.

    EXTREMITIES: Unremarkable. Pulses strong and equal.

    LABORATORY DATA: Hemoglobin, 12.3. White count, 10.800. Normal electrolytes. ECG shows sinus bradycardia.

DIAGNOSIS: Weakness on the basis of sinus bradycardia, probably Cardizem induced.

TREATMENT: Patient told to change positions slowly when moving from sitting to standing, and from lying to standing.

John R. Ramirez, MD

Figure 2-1 Example of Physical Examination Documentation

Jennifer Delgado
8/14/2008

SUBJECTIVE: The patient has had epilepsy since she was 10. She takes her medication as prescribed; denies side effects. She reports no convulsions or new symptoms. She is a full-time student at Riverside Community College.

OBJECTIVE: Phenobarbital 90 mg twice a day as prescribed since 1994. The motor and sensory examination results are normal.

ASSESSMENT: Well-controlled epilepsy.

PLAN: Patient advised to continue medication regimen. Schedule for follow-up in 6 months.

Jared R. Wandaowsky, MD

Figure 2-2 Example of a Progress Note

Every patient visit should be documented with the following information:
- The patient's name
- The encounter date and reason
- Appropriate history and physical examination
- Review of all tests that were ordered
- The diagnosis
- The plan of care, or notes on treatments that were given
- The instructions or recommendations that were given to the patient
- The signature of the provider who saw the patient.

In addition to this encounter information, a patient's medical record must contain:
- Biographical and personal information, including the patient's full name, Social Security number, date of birth, full address, marital status, home and work telephone numbers, and employer information as applicable
- Duplicates of all documents that communicate with the patient, including letters, telephone calls, faxes, and e-mail messages; the patient's responses; and a note of the time, date, topic, and physician's response to each communication from the patient
- Duplicates of prescriptions and instructions given to the patient, including refills

- Any original documents that the patient has signed, such as an authorization to release information (see page 26) and an advance directive
- Medical allergies and reactions, or the lack of them
- Up-to-date immunization record and history if appropriate, such as for a child
- Previous and current diagnoses, test results, health risks, and progress
- Copies of referral or consultation letters
- Hospital admissions and release documents
- A record of any missed or canceled appointments
- Any requests for information about the patient (from a health plan or an attorney, for example), and a detailed log of to whom information was released

The patient medical record also includes the identification number assigned by the practice to the patient. Billing and insurance information is usually stored separately from the medical record.

PROTECTED HEALTH INFORMATION AND MEDICAL RECORDS

Health is a personal and private matter. Patients may share health information with physicians that could change their lives or cause them to lose a job or friends. Nevertheless, medical information must be recorded in medical records and communicated to others in the course of treatment and payment.

HIPAA Privacy Rule

To ensure that health information is protected from misuse, a federal law, the Health Insurance Portability and Accountability Act, or HIPAA (pronounced hip-uh), regulates how electronic patient information is stored and shared. Part of this act, the HIPAA Privacy Rule, must be followed by health plans, health care clearinghouses, and health care providers, as well as by the outside businesses that work with them, such as medical billing companies and accounting firms.

Protected Health Information

The Privacy Rule establishes the definition of each patient's protected health information (PHI). PHI is any individually identifiable health information that is transmitted or maintained by electronic media, such as sent over the Internet or stored in the office's computer files. Under this definition, a report of the number of people treated by a physician who have diabetes is not PHI, but the names of the patients are protected. PHI includes many facts about people, such as names, addresses, birth dates, employers, telephone numbers, Social Security numbers, and health plan beneficiary numbers, any of which could be used to identify them.

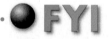

FYI

A **clearinghouse** is a company that helps medical offices and health plans exchange claim data in correct formats. Clearinghouses, for instance, are able to accept paper claims from a physician and transform them to electronic claims that are HIPAA compliant.

Privacy Practices

The Privacy Rule also sets out the things that medical offices must do to properly handle patients' PHI:

- The practice must adopt privacy practices that are appropriate for its health care services.
- The practice must notify patients about their privacy rights and how their information may be used or disclosed.
- Office employees must be trained so that they understand the privacy practices.
- A staff member must be appointed as the office's privacy official and be responsible for seeing that privacy practices are adopted and followed.
- Patients' records containing individually identifiable health information must be maintained and stored so that they are not readily available to those who do not need them.

Notice of and Acknowledgment of Receipt of Notice of Privacy Practices

To comply with the Privacy Rule, medical offices, as well as other providers and health plans, must give each patient an explanation of privacy practices at the patient's first contact or encounter. To satisfy this requirement, medical offices give patients a copy of their Notice of Privacy Practices (see Figure 2-3 on pages 28–29). The notice explains how patients' PHI may be used and describes their rights. The office must also ask patients to review this notice and sign an Acknowledgment of Receipt of Notice of Privacy Practices, showing that they have read and understand the document (see Figure 2-4 on page 30).

Sharing Protected Health Information

The Privacy Rule recognizes that medical offices and payers must be able to exchange PHI in the normal course of business. The rule says that there are three everyday situations in which PHI can be released *without* the patient's permission: treatment, payment, and operations (**TPO**).

- *Treatment* means providing and coordinating the patient's medical care. Physicians and other medical staff members can discuss patients' cases in the office and with other physicians. Laboratory or X-ray technicians may call to clarify requests they cannot read because of the physician's handwriting. This information can be provided by the physician or another medical staff member.
- *Payment* refers to the exchange of information with health plans. Medical office staff members can take the required information from patients' records and prepare health care claims that are transmitted to health plans.
- *Operations* are the general business management functions needed to run the office.

Central Practice Center

NOTICE OF PRIVACY PRACTICES

THIS NOTICE DESCRIBES HOW MEDICAL INFORMATION ABOUT YOU MAY BE USED AND DISCLOSED AND HOW YOU CAN GET ACCESS TO THIS INFORMATION. PLEASE REVIEW IT CAREFULLY.

WHY ARE YOU GETTING THIS NOTICE?

Central Practice Center is required by federal and state law to maintain the privacy of your health information. The use and disclosure of your health information is governed by regulations under the Health Insurance Portability and Accountability Act of 1996 (HIPAA) and the requirements of applicable state law. For health information covered by HIPAA, we are required to provide you with this Notice and will abide by this Notice with respect to such health information. If you have questions about this Notice, please contact our Privacy Officer at 877-555-1313. We will ask you to sign an "acknowledgment" indicating that you have been provided with this notice.

WHAT HEALTH INFORMATION IS PROTECTED?

We are committed to protecting the privacy of information we gather about you while providing health-related services. Some examples of protected health information are:

- Information indicating that you are a patient receiving treatment or other health-related services from our physicians or staff;
- Information about your health condition (such as a disease you may have);
- Information about health care products or services you have received or may receive in the future (such as an operation); or
- Information about your health care benefits under an insurance plan (such as whether a prescription is covered);

when combined with:

- Demographic information (such as your name, address, or insurance status);
- Unique numbers that may identify you (such as your Social Security number, your phone number, or your driver's license number); and
- Other types of information that may identify who you are.

SUMMARY OF THIS NOTICE

This summary includes references to paragraphs throughout this notice that you may read for additional information.

1. Written Authorization Requirement

We may use your health information or share it with others in order to treat your condition, obtain payment for that treatment, and run our business operations. We generally need your written authorization for other uses and disclosures of your health information, unless an exception described in this Notice applies.

2. Authorizing Transfer of Your Records

You may request that we transfer your records to another person or organization by completing a written authorization form. This form will specify what information is being released, to whom, and for what purpose. The authorization will have an expiration date.

3. Canceling Your Written Authorization

If you provide us with written authorization, you may revoke, or cancel, it at any time, except to the extent that we have already relied upon it. To revoke a written authorization, please write to the doctor's office where you initially gave your authorization.

4. Exceptions to Written Authorization Requirement

There are some situations in which we do not need your written authorization before using your health information or sharing it with others. They include:

Treatment, Payment and Operations
As mentioned above, we may use your health information or share it with others in order to treat your condition, obtain payment for that treatment, and run our business operations.

Family and Friends
If you do not object, we will share information about your health with family and friends involved in your care.

Figure 2-3a Example of a Notice of Privacy Practices

Research
Although we will generally try to obtain your written authorization before using your health information for research purposes, there may be certain situations in which we are not required to obtain your written authorization.

De-Identified Information
We may use or disclose your health information if we have removed any information that might identify you. When all identifying information is removed, we say that the health information is "completely de-identified." We may also use and disclose "partially de-identified" information if the person who will receive it agrees in writing to protect your privacy when using the information.

Incidental Disclosures
We may inadvertently use or disclose your health information despite having taken all reasonable precautions to protect the privacy and confidentiality of your health information.

Emergencies or Public Need
We may use or disclose your health information in an emergency or for important public health needs. For example, we may share your information with public health officials at the State or city health departments who are authorized to investigate and control the spread of diseases.

5. How to Access Your Health Information

You generally have the right to inspect and get copies of your health information.

6. How to Correct Your Health Information

You have the right to request that we amend your health information if you believe it is inaccurate or incomplete.

7. How to Identify Others Who Have Received Your Health Information

You have the right to receive an "accounting of disclosures." This is a report that identifies certain persons or organizations to which we have disclosed your health information. All disclosures are made according to the protections described in this Notice of Privacy Practices. Many routine disclosures we make (for treatment, payment, or business operations, among others) will not be included in this report. However, it will identify any non-routine disclosures of your information.

8. How to Request Additional Privacy Protections

You have the right to request further restrictions on the way we use your health information or share it with others. However, we are not required to agree to the restriction you request. If we do agree with your request, we will be bound by our agreement.

9. How to Request Alternative Communications

You have the right to request that we contact you in a way that is more confidential for you, such as at home instead of at work. We will try to accommodate all reasonable requests.

10. How Someone May Act On Your Behalf

You have the right to name a personal representative who may act on your behalf to control the privacy of your health information. Parents and guardians will generally have the right to control the privacy of health information about minors unless the minors are permitted by law to act on their own behalf.

11. How to Learn about Special Protections for HIV, Alcohol and Substance Abuse, Mental Health and Genetic Information

Special privacy protections apply to HIV-related information, alcohol and substance abuse treatment information, mental health information, psychotherapy notes and genetic information.

12. How to Obtain A Copy of This Notice

If you have not already received one, you have the right to a paper copy of this notice. You may request a paper copy at any time, even if you have previously agreed to receive this notice electronically. You can request a copy of the privacy notice directly from your doctor's office. You may also obtain a copy of this notice from our website or by requesting a copy at your next visit.

13. How to Obtain A Copy of Revised Notice

We may change our privacy practices from time to time. If we do, we will revise this notice so you will have an accurate summary of our practices. You will be able to obtain your own copy of the revised notice by accessing our website or by calling your doctor's office. You may also ask for one at the time of your next visit. The effective date of the notice is noted in the top right corner of each page. We are required to abide by the terms of the notice that is currently in effect.

14. How To File A Complaint

If you believe your privacy rights have been violated, you may file a complaint with us or with the federal Office of Civil Rights. To file a complaint with us, please contact our Privacy Officer.

No one will retaliate or take action against you for filing a complaint.

Figure 2-3b Example of a Notice of Privacy Practices (*cont.*)

Acknowledgment of Receipt of Notice of Privacy Practices

I understand that the providers of Central Practice Center may share my health information for treatment, billing and healthcare operations. I have been given a copy of the organization's notice of privacy practices that describes how my health information is used and shared. I understand that Central Practice Center has the right to change this notice at any time. I may obtain a current copy by contacting the practice's office or by visiting the website at www.xxx.com.

My signature below constitutes my acknowledgment that I have been provided with a copy of the notice of privacy practices.

_____

Signature of Patient or Legal Representative   Date

If signed by legal representative,
relationship to patient:_____

Figure 2-4 Example of an Acknowledgment of Receipt of Notice of Privacy Practices

Minimum Necessary Standard

When using protected health information, a medical office must try to limit the information shared to the minimum amount of PHI necessary to accomplish the intended purpose. The minimum necessary standard means taking reasonable safeguards to protect PHI from incidental disclosure. For example, a medical insurance specialist would not disclose a patient's history of cancer on a workers' compensation claim for a sprained ankle. Only the information the recipient needs to know is given.

Avoid using fax transmissions for confidential information, because they are hard to protect. If electronic transmission, such as e-mail, is used to send a patient's information, be sure to carefully follow the medical office's guidelines for Internet security.

Professional Focus

Office of Civil Rights

Patients who observe privacy problems in their providers' offices can complain either to the medical office or to the Department of Health and Human Services (HHS). Complaints must be put in writing, on paper or electronically, and sent to the **Office of Civil Rights** **(OCR),** which is part of HHS, usually within 180 days. The office must cooperate with an HHS investigation and give HHS access to its facilities, books, records, and systems, including relevant protected health information.

HIPAA Tip

Medical insurance specialists should be careful not to discuss patients' cases with anyone outside the office, including family and friends. Avoid talking about cases, too, in the practice's reception areas, where other patients might overhear comments. Close charts on desks when they are not being worked on. A computer screen displaying a patient's records should be positioned so that only the person working with the file can view it. Files should be closed when the computer is not in use.

Authorizations

For use or disclosure of PHI other than for treatment, payment, or operations (TPO), the patient must sign an authorization to release the information. For example, information about alcohol and drug abuse may not be released without a specific authorization from the patient. The authorization document must be in plain language and include the following:

- A description of the information to be used or disclosed
- The name or other specific identification of the person(s) authorized to use or disclose the information
- The name of the person(s) or group of people to whom the covered entity may make the disclosure
- A description of the purpose of each requested use or disclosure.
- An expiration date
- Signature of the individual (or authorized representative) and date

A sample authorization form is shown in Figure 2-5 on page 32.

Patients have the right to an accounting of disclosures of their PHI other than for treatment, payment, or operations purposes. The medical office keeps a disclosure log for each patient, so that authorized disclosures can be listed. When an accidental disclosure of a patient's PHI occurs, it should also be documented in the individual's medical record, since it did not fall into a permitted disclosure purpose for TPO, and the individual did not authorize the disclosure. An example is sending a consultation report to the wrong physician's office.

HIPAA Tip

To legally release PHI for purposes other than treatment, payment, or health care operations, a signed authorization document is required.

Exceptions to the Privacy Rule

There are a number of exceptions to the privacy rule. All these types of disclosures must also be logged, and the release information must be available to the patient who requests it.

- *Release Under Court Order*—If the patient's PHI is required as evidence by a court of law, the provider may release it without the patient's approval upon judicial order. In the case of a lawsuit, a court sometimes decides that a physician or medical practice staff member must provide testimony. The court issues a subpoena, an

Case Study

Medical information must be kept confidential, even in a moral dilemma. For example, a woman with a sexually transmitted disease has identified John as one of her sexual partners. John came into the office and began receiving treatment with an antibiotic. Then, one day, John's wife, Marsha, received billing notices and called to ask whether there had been a billing error. Near tears and frightened, Marsha pleads, "Why is he seeing the doctor? Can't you tell me what's wrong with my husband?" The medical insurance specialist is caught in a moral dilemma. It appears that John has not told Marsha about his disease, despite the fact that she most likely will contract the infection.

The medical insurance specialist cannot release John's protected health information, even in this case. In responding to Marsha, the correct thing to say is, "I cannot disclose patient information. Why don't you discuss the bill with your husband?"

Patient Name: _____

Health Record Number: _____

Date of Birth: _____

1. I authorize the use or disclosure of the above named individual's health information as described below.

2. The following individual(s) or organization(s) are authorized to make the disclosure: _____

3. The type of information to be used or disclosed is as follows (check the appropriate boxes and include other information where indicated)
❑ problem list
❑ medication list
❑ list of allergies
❑ immunization records
❑ most recent history
❑ most recent discharge summary
❑ lab results (please describe the dates or types of lab tests you would like disclosed): _____
❑ x-ray and imaging reports (please describe the dates or types of x-rays or images you
    would like disclosed): _____
❑ consultation reports from (please supply doctors' names): _____
❑ entire record
❑ other (please describe): _____

4. I understand that the information in my health record may include information relating to sexually transmitted disease, acquired immunodeficiency syndrome (AIDS), or human immunodeficiency virus (HIV). It may also include information about behavioral or mental health services, and treatment for alcohol and drug abuse.

5. The information identified above may be used by or disclosed to the following individuals or organization(s):

Name: _____

Address: _____

Name: _____

Address: _____

6. This information for which I'm authorizing disclosure will be used for the following purpose:
❑ my personal records
❑ sharing with other health care providers as needed/other (please describe): _____

7. I understand that I have a right to revoke this authorization at any time. I understand that if I revoke this authorization, I must do so in writing and present my written revocation to the health information management department. I understand that the revocation will not apply to information that has already been released in response to this authorization. I understand that the revocation will not apply to my insurance company when the law provides my insurer with the right to contest a claim under my policy.

8. This authorization will expire (insert date or event): _____

If I fail to specify an expiration date or event, this authorization will expire six months
from the date on which it was signed.

9. I understand that once the above information is disclosed, it may be redisclosed by the recipient and the information may not be protected by federal privacy laws or regulations.

10. I understand authorizing the use or disclosure of the information identified above is voluntary. I need not sign this form to ensure healthcare treatment.

Signature of patient or legal representative: _____ Date: _____

If signed by legal representative, relationship to patient

Signature of witness: _____ Date: _____

Distribution of copies: Original to provider; copy to patient; copy to accompany use or disclosure

Note: This sample form was developed by the American Health Information Management Association for discussion purposes. It should not be used without review by the issuing organization's legal counsel to ensure compliance with other federal and state laws and regulations.

What specific information can be released

To whom

For what purpose

Figure 2-5 Example of an Authorization to Use or Disclose Health Information

order of the court directing a party to appear and testify. If the court requires the witness to bring certain evidence, such as a patient's medical record, it issues a subpoena *duces tecum*, which directs the party to appear, to testify, and to bring specified documents or items.

- *Workers' Compensation Cases*—State law may provide for release of records to employers in workers' compensation cases (see Chapter 12). The law may also authorize release to the state workers' compensation administration board and to the insurance company that handles these claims for the state.

- *Statutory Reports*—Some specific types of information are required by state law to be released to state health or social services departments. For example, physicians must make such statutory reports for patients' births and deaths and for cases of abuse. Because of the danger of harm to patients or others, communicable diseases such as tuberculosis, hepatitis, and rabies must usually be reported.

- *HIV and AIDS*—A special category of communicable disease control is applied to patients with diagnoses of human immunodeficiency virus (HIV) infection and acquired immunodeficiency syndrome (AIDS). Every state requires AIDS cases to be reported. Most states also require reporting of the HIV infection that causes the syndrome. However, state law varies concerning whether only the fact of a case is to be reported, or if the patient's name must also be reported. The medical office's guidelines will reflect the state laws and must be strictly observed, as all these regulations should be, to protect patients' privacy and to comply with the regulations.

- *Research Data*—PHI may be made available to researchers approved by the practice. For example, if a physician is conducting clinical research on a type of diabetes, the practice may share information from appropriate records for analysis. When the researcher issues reports or studies based on the information, specific patients' names may not be identified.

- *De-Identified Health Information*—There are no restrictions on the use or disclosure of "de-identified" health information that does not identify an individual.

RECORD RETENTION

Each medical office develops a retention schedule to control how long patient information is stored. The retention schedule is based on the law of the state and, if the office sees Medicare or Medicaid patients, federal regulations. The guidelines cover what information should be kept, for how long, and in what storage medium, such as paper, microfilm, or computer files. If records are to be destroyed at some point after retention, the means of disposal is also covered in the guidelines.

Medical records have a high degree of credibility because the law assumes that patients state only true information to their physicians. A medical office's financial records can be audited for up to seven years from a patient's last visit, and for a longer period if embezzlement of government funds has occurred. Patients' medical records, on the other hand, should be maintained indefinitely if an account is contested or if there is a possibility that a patient's illness may not be resolved.

The physician documents critical patient–physician events in the patient's medical record. For example, a physician who is withdrawing from a case usually states in writing the patient's status and confirms that he or she is not doing further work. If a patient does not follow the treatment plan, the physician should document this in writing with a copy of the letter to the patient. This information is maintained in the patient's file. Depending on the physician's policy, if a patient has not returned for medical care after seven years, the records can be destroyed. Medical offices have written procedures that cover how long records are retained and what method is used to destroy them at the proper time.

AVOIDING FRAUD

Fraud occurs when someone intentionally misrepresents facts to receive a benefit illegally. A person who cooperates in a fraudulent situation is also personally responsible. In a medical office, some of the most common fraudulent situations include:

- Altering the patient's chart to increase the amount reimbursed.
- Upgrading or falsifying medical procedures to increase the amount reimbursed.
- Overbilling primary and secondary insurance carriers while at the same time collecting payment from the patient.

Fraud and HIPAA

HIPAA clearly defines health care fraud as a crime. The act set up the Health Care Fraud and Abuse Control Program to coordinate federal, state, and local law enforcement through investigations, audits, evaluations, and inspections. This program is not limited to Medicare and Medicaid. It covers any plan or program that provides health benefits, such as health insurance policies. When fraud is determined, the law permits fines of up to $10,000 per item or service for which fraudulent payment was received. Criminal penalties—fines and imprisonment—exist for knowingly planning to obtain money or property owned by the health care benefit program. If a patient is seriously hurt because of a fraudulent act, a guilty person can be imprisoned for up to twenty years. Life imprisonment is possible if the violation results in a patient's death.

Only physicians who are in clinical practice can prescribe medications. For example, doctors in research cannot write prescriptions. Furthermore, to dispense narcotic drugs, the physician must register with the Drug Enforcement Administration and receive a permit. In the medical office, all drugs and prescription pads must be locked away. Concerns about the way drugs are stored should be reported to the office manager or the physician.

Knowingly is a key word in fraud cases. Most physicians maintain an honest relationship with insurance carriers. Some, however, do not. For example, suppose a physician asks a staff member to code a patient's headaches as a subdural hematoma (pool of blood below the dura mater membrane of the brain) in order to justify billing an expensive procedure. An employee must never falsify medical records. Here is what can happen: The physician might receive the higher payment, but the federal government audits the records of the medical office, finds that the patient's record does not match the insurance claim, and successfully prosecutes the physician and the staff member, finding the staff member responsible.

Professional Focus

COMPLIANCE PLANS

Under federal law, the Office of Inspector General (OIG) is responsible for investigating suspected health care fraud. So that physicians can take steps to prevent the submission of erroneous claims or other unlawful conduct, the OIG has issued the Compliance Program for Individual and Small Group Physician Practices. This program outlines the parts of a **compliance plan** that each medical office should write and then communicate to staff. An effective program has these parts:

(1) conducting audits and monitoring how well the medical office follows the applicable rules, (2) implementing compliance and practice standards, (3) appointing a compliance officer on staff, (4) conducting appropriate staff training, (5) responding appropriately to fix problems that are found, (6) making sure that employees can communicate openly if they think there are compliance problems, and (7) enforcing the standards and publicizing the rules in the medical office.

The Medical Insurance Specialist's Role

Avoid becoming accidentally involved in fraud by making sure all insurance information is true. A diagnosis or procedure code must not be added to any insurance claim if the information is not documented in the patient's record by the physician. If the medical insurance specialist suspects that something has been mistakenly left out, the physician should be asked to update the record before the information is entered on the claim.

Because of their contracts with physicians, many health plans have the right to audit the physician's billing practices. Sometimes carriers audit selected physicians because they provide extraordinary or very specialized services. Other audits are conducted in cases where fraud or other misrepresentation of services is suspected. The health plan will notify the physician before an audit is conducted, and the types of records that will be audited are specified ahead of time. The role of the medical insurance specialist is to make sure the records are available, complete, and signed by the physician.

Chapter Summary

1. Patients' medical records, which contain the complete, chronological, and comprehensive documentation of patients' health history and status, are used by providers to communicate and coordinate patients' health care. The records are used by medical insurance specialists to prepare and support insurance claims. If it is not documented, a service should not be billed.

2. Patients' protected health information (PHI) is defined as individually identifiable health information that is transmitted or maintained by electronic media. HIPAA requires medical offices to observe a number of regulations in order to protect the use and disclosure of PHI.

3. The HIPAA Privacy Rule regulates the use and disclosure of PHI. It requires medical offices to have a Notice of Privacy Practices, for example, and also to give patients this notice.

4. For use or disclosure for treatment, payment, or operations (TPO), no release is required from the patient.

5. To release PHI for other than TPO, a medical office must have the patient sign an authorization. The authorization document must be in plain language and have a description of the information to be used, who can disclose it and for what purpose, who will receive it, an expiration date, and the patient's signature.

6. A retention schedule provides guidelines on the items in the patient's medical record that must be retained and on the length of time for retention. Also, the provider must be able to justify the level and nature of treatment when a claim is investigated or challenged.

7. To protect against potential fraud, the medical practice should have a compliance plan in place. Medical insurance specialists must observe the appropriate rules about release of patient information and about correct coding and billing.

Check Your Understanding

Part 1. Write "T" or "F" in the blank to indicate whether you think the statement is true or false.

F **1.** Medical office staff members are free to share information about patients with their families and friends.

T **2.** Health care fraud is a crime.

F **3.** Reporting services that were not performed to improve cash flow is an acceptable practice.

T **4.** The medical record must contain documentation that supports a billed service.

FT **5.** The HIPAA law is different in each state.

TF **6.** The minimum necessary standard helps to determine what PHI should be shared.

T **7.** Under the HIPAA Privacy Rule, patients' protected health information can be released to payers for payment purposes.

T **8.** A retention schedule does not apply to clinical records.

F **9.** The authorization to use and disclose medical information form authorizes the sharing of all confidential information with the patient's family members.

T **10.** Information about a patient should never be released over the telephone without being sure that the inquirer is entitled to it.

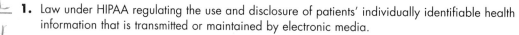

Part 2. Match each term below with its correct definition.

- **A.** HIPAA Privacy Rule
- **B.** authorization
- **C.** minimum necessary standard
- **D.** fraud
- **E.** clearinghouse
- **F.** Notice of Privacy Practices
- **G.** compliance plan
- **H.** subpoena
- **I.** retention schedule
- **J.** PHI

A **1.** Law under HIPAA regulating the use and disclosure of patients' individually identifiable health information that is transmitted or maintained by electronic media.

H **2.** An order to appear or produce something in court.

C **3.** The principle that individually identifiable health information should be disclosed only to the extent needed to support the purpose of the disclosure.

F **4.** A HIPAA-mandated document that presents a medical office's principles and procedures related to the protection of patients' protected health information.

E **5.** A company that offers providers, for a fee, the service of receiving electronic or paper claims, checking and preparing them for processing, and transmitting them in proper data format to the correct carriers.

B **6.** Document signed by a patient that permits release of medical information under the specific stated conditions.

G **7.** A medical practice's written plan that includes auditing and monitoring compliance with government regulations, developing consistent written policies and procedures, providing ongoing staff training and communication, and responding to and correcting errors.

D **8.** A wrongdoing, or misconduct.

J **9.** Any information about a patient that might be used to identify the person, such as name, address, or Social Security number.

I **10.** An office policy governing the information from patients' medical records that is to be stored, for how long it is to be retained, and the storage medium to be used.

Part 3. Classify each of the following situations as fraudulent (F), acceptable practice (A), or a violation of the HIPAA Privacy Rule (V).

F **1.** A medical insurance specialist alters a Medicare patient's claim by coding a service that was not performed.

A **2.** The physician tells a nurse about a patient's diagnosis.

V **3.** The medical practice's receptionist discusses a patient's diagnosis with a friend.

A **4.** A patient tells a physician personal details about an old condition unrelated to the current diagnosis.

A **5.** A medical office files a report with the state authority regarding births and deaths among the practice's patients in the past year.

___V___ **6.** A medical office handling a workers' compensation case tells the patient's employer about his history of skin cancer.

___A∅___ **7.** A primary care physician sends information to a referred specialist without an authorization.

___A___ **8.** A medical insurance specialist supplies information about a patient to the patient's insurance carrier.

___E___ **9.** The physician performs five services that were not medically necessary.

___E___**10.** A medical insurance specialist submits a Medicare claim form that bills for noncovered services.

Part 4. **The X-ray report below contains four documentation errors. Identify each, and indicate the guideline that has not been followed.**

X-RAY REPORT

Patient name
Salvia, Leonard X.

Examination
Esophagus

Report

Just put line through it. *mu 7-20-05* *jdl 7-20-2005*

① The patient experiences no difficulty in swallowing barium. A ~~2~~ cm tablet was given and

② passes readily down to the distal esophagus. After considerable swallowing, the barium

③ tablet remained in place, indicating a significant area of narrowing, less than 1 cm in

④ diameter, located between this distal esophagus that probably represents a stricture related

⑤ to a small hiatus hernia and possible esophagitis. There are no shelf-like defects or masses   *Jane jm 7-20-05*

⑥ to correspond to neoplasm. The mid and upper ~~position~~ *portion* of the esophagus is unremarkable.

⑦ Conclusion: Small hiatus hernia with an area of stenosis, probably on the basis of

⑧ esophagitis, appears to represent a ~~significant~~ *major* lesion.   *jm 7-20-05*   *jdl*

Objectives

After completing this chapter, you will be able to define the key terms and:

1. Explain how diagnostic coding affects the payment process.
2. Label the primary diagnosis and coexisting conditions.
3. Explain the ICD format, and identify sections used by medical insurance specialists in physician practices.
4. Identify the purpose and correct use of V codes and E codes.
5. Use a five-step process to analyze diagnoses and locate the correct ICD code.

Key Terms

Alphabetic Index
category
chief complaint (CC)
coexisting condition
conventions
cross-reference
diagnosis code

Dx
E code
etiology
*International Classification of
    Diseases*, Ninth Revision,
    Clinical Modification (ICD)
main term

primary diagnosis
subcategory
subclassification
subterm
supplementary term
Tabular List
V code

Why This Chapter Is Important to You

The information in this chapter will enable you to:
- Use an important reference book, the ICD-9-CM.
- Expand your understanding of why errors in diagnostic coding interfere with the billing and payment cycle.
- Learn one of the most important steps in completing health care claims.

What Do You Think?

To diagnose a patient's condition, the physician follows a complex process of decision making based on the patient's statements, an examination, and evaluation of this information. When the diagnosis is made, the medical insurance specialist communicates it to the insurance carrier through codes on the health care claim. What impact does incorrect coding have on the medical office?

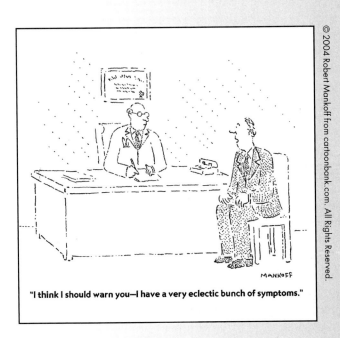

"I think I should warn you—I have a very eclectic bunch of symptoms."

INTRODUCTION TO DIAGNOSTIC CODING

During the course of office encounters (visits) with patients, physicians document their evaluations of patients' conditions in their medical records. For example, in a section called Review of Systems (ROS), the patient's responses to the physician's questions about each body system are recorded. When an examination is conducted, physicians summarize the findings under various headings, such as "neck" or "neurologic" (for the nervous system). Patients' medical records also include treatments, progress notes, follow-up care, laboratory and X-ray reports, and special forms.

When a diagnosis is made by the physician, it is documented in the patient's medical record. The diagnosis, often abbreviated **Dx** in the medical record, describes illnesses or injuries using medical terminology. Medical insurance specialists become familiar with the most common diagnoses of patients seen in their medical offices. For example, in a cardiologist's office, terms such as *hypertension, cardiac infarction, vascular disease, coronary stenosis,* and *angina pectoris* are typical of the medical terminology used to describe a variety of heart conditions. Regardless of the type of medical practice, all diagnoses can be indicated by a coded "language" that is recognized worldwide.

Diagnosis Codes

One of the most important pieces of information on a health care claim is the diagnosis. The code number entered there is based on the physician's opinion of the patient's specific illness(es), sign(s), symptom(s), and complaint(s). This number is the diagnosis code.

Coding affects the medical billing and payment process. Diagnosis codes give insurance carriers clearly defined diagnoses to help process claims efficiently. An error in coding conveys to an insurance carrier the wrong reason a patient received medical services. This causes confusion, a delay in processing, and possibly a reduced payment or denial of the claim. An incorrect code may also raise the question of fraudulent billing if the payer decides that, based on the diagnosis, the services provided were not medically necessary.

The ICD-9-CM

The diagnosis codes are found in the International Classification of Diseases, Ninth Revision, Clinical Modification, referred to as the ICD. The ICD is a single book or set of multiple volumes that lists codes according to a system assigned by the World Health Organization of the United Nations. The volumes are distributed by the United States Government Printing Office in Washington, D.C., and by commercial publishers.

The ICD had its beginnings in England in the 1600s. By the late 1800s it was used in the United States for reporting morbidity (the prevalence of an illness) and mortality (causes of death) statistics. Today, computers collect and analyze ICD codes used by government health care programs, professional standards review organizations, medical researchers, hospitals, physicians, and other health care providers. Private and public medical insurance carriers also use the codes.

The ICD has been revised a number of times. ICD-9, for example, refers to the ninth revision of the ICD. In the title, ICD-9-CM, the initials *CM* indicate that the edition is a clinical modification. For example, the ICD-9-CM is the clinical modification of the ninth revision of the ICD. Codes in this modification describe various conditions and illnesses with more precision than did earlier codes. Under HIPAA, ICD-9-CM codes must be used to report diagnoses on all claims.

The coding system in the ICD-9-CM contains three-digit categories for diseases, injuries, and symptoms. Almost all of these three-digit categories are divided into four-digit code groups called subcategories. Many are further divided into five-digit codes called subclassifications. In the ICD-9-CM, the fourth and fifth digits are separated from the first three by a period. The purpose of the fourth- and fifth-level diagnosis codes is to permit reporting the most specific diagnosis possible. Figure 3-1 shows an example of several levels of ICD codes.

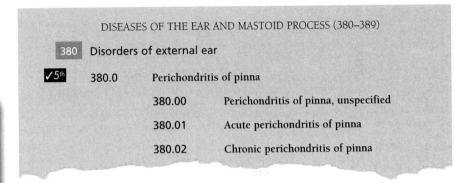

DISEASES OF THE EAR AND MASTOID PROCESS (380–389)

380	Disorders of external ear	
✓5th	380.0	Perichondritis of pinna
	380.00	Perichondritis of pinna, unspecified
	380.01	Acute perichondritis of pinna
	380.02	Chronic perichondritis of pinna

Figure 3-1 Examples of the Three Levels of ICD Codes

In addition to the categories for diseases, one section of the ICD-9-CM codes begins with the letter *V,* and another section begins with *E.* These letters are followed by up to four digits. The codes that begin with *V* are used for encounters for reasons other than illness or injury. In these situations, patients often do not have a complaint or active diagnosis. For example, a routine annual physical examination is a reason for an office visit without a complaint. Visits for treatments of a diagnosed condition, such as chemotherapy for cancer, also receive codes beginning with *V.* Codes beginning with *E* indicate the external cause of an injury or poisoning. For example, a patient's harmful reaction to the proper dosage of a drug is assigned an E code. Both types of codes are described in more detail later in this chapter.

CODING BASICS FOR PHYSICIAN PRACTICES

A health care claim for a patient must show the diagnosis that represents the patient's major health problem *for that particular encounter.* This condition is the primary diagnosis. The primary diagnosis must provide the reason for medical services listed on that claim. If a patient has cancer, for example, the disease is probably the patient's major health problem. However, if that patient sees the physician for an ear infection that is not related to the cancer, the primary diagnosis for that particular claim is the ear infection.

At times, there is more than one diagnosis because many patients are treated by a health care provider for more than one illness. Someone with hypertension (high blood pressure), for example, may also have heart disease. A patient with diabetes may seek care for a respiratory infection. The primary diagnosis—the underlying condition—is listed first on the insurance claim. After that, additional coexisting condition(s) may be listed. Coexisting conditions occur at the same time as the primary diagnosis and affect the treatment or recovery from the condition shown as the primary diagnosis. For example, a patient with diabetes mellitus often suffers from poor circulation. The diagnosis for this person's office visit to complain of numbness in the fingers and toes would be likely to include the diabetes as a coexisting condition. Sometimes, a diagnosis code contains both the primary and a coexisting condition. For example, code 365.63 means glaucoma associated with vascular disorders.

Examples

The information for identifying a patient's diagnosis and any coexisting conditions is found in the patient's medical record. When the patient goes into the examining room, a medical assistant or nurse may conduct a short interview to find out the patient's chief complaint (abbreviated CC in the documentation). The chief complaint is the reason the patient seeks medical care on this encounter. Notes about the chief complaint may be entered in the patient's medical record by the medical assistant, nurse, or physician. However, *only* the physician determines the diagnosis.

Suppose Rosa Hernandez, a patient, comes to the office. Notes about the encounter might appear as follows:

CC: Diarrhea X 5 days with strong odor and mucus, abdominal pain and tenderness, no meds.
Dx: Ulcerative colitis.

The notes mean that Ms. Hernandez has had symptoms for five days and has taken no medication. Her chief complaint is noted after the abbreviation *CC*. Her diagnosis, listed after the abbreviation *Dx*, is ulcerative colitis.

Now suppose another patient, Joel Perlman, sees the physician. His record indicates a history of heavy smoking and includes an X-ray report and notes such as these:

CC: Hoarseness, pain during swallowing, dyspnea during exertion.
Dx: Emphysema and laryngitis.

The physician listed emphysema, the major health problem, first. It is Mr. Perlman's primary diagnosis. Laryngitis is a coexisting condition that is being treated.

Finally, a third patient, Janet Chang, has a prior history of breast cancer. For today's visit, her progress notes read:

CC: Laceration of right great toe three days previously, experiencing pain, toe reddened and swollen.
Dx: Complicated open wound of toe.

Ms. Chang's primary diagnosis for this encounter is a complicated open wound of the toe. The cancer is not reported on the health care claim because the physician has not stated that it affects Ms. Chang's recovery time and or the way the wound is treated.

682.6 (handwritten)

Case Study 3-1

Patient: Hector Garcia
  CC: Red swollen lump on thigh noticed four days ago; became painful today.
  Dx: Abscess.

682.6 (handwritten)

What is Hector Garcia's primary diagnosis?
Answer: _Abscess_ (handwritten)

Case Study 3-2

Patient: James Jacobson
  CC: Left-knee pain, swelling, and weakness. Has had right-knee pain and arthritis in past.
  Dx: Left-knee pain and swelling secondary to gouty arthritis.

274.0 (handwritten)

What is James Jacobson's primary diagnosis?
Answer: _gouty arthritis_ (handwritten)

USING THE ICD

As mentioned earlier, the ICD comes in the form of a single book or a set of two or three books. Three sections are available:

Volume 1—Diseases: Tabular List
Volume 2—Diseases: Alphabetic Index
Volume 3—Procedures: Tabular List and Alphabetic Index

Notice that the ICD covers two major areas, diseases and procedures. Medical insurance specialists in a medical office use only the diagnosis codes (Volumes 1 and 2) in the ICD. The procedures (Volume 3) are used only for hospital tests and treatments. Use of Volume 3 is covered in Chapter 15 of this text.

In the ICD, diagnoses are listed two ways, as illustrated in Figure 3-2 on page 46. One is the Alphabetic Index, which lists diagnoses in alphabetic order with their corresponding diagnosis codes. The other is the Tabular List, which provides diagnosis codes in numerical order with additional instructions.

Both the Alphabetic Index and the Tabular List are used to find the right code. The Alphabetic Index is never used alone, because it does not contain all the necessary information. After a code is located in the Alphabetic Index, it is looked up in the Tabular List. Notes in this list may suggest or require the use of additional codes. Alternatively, notes may indicate that conditions should be coded differently because of exclusion from a category.

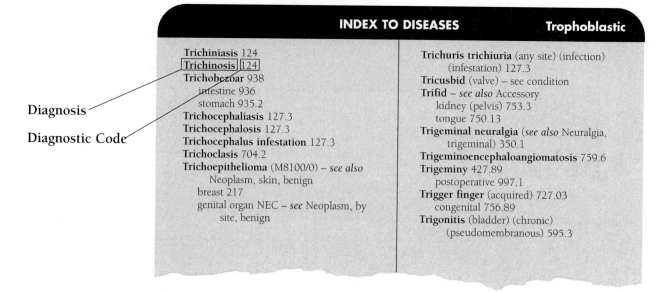

Alphabetic Index

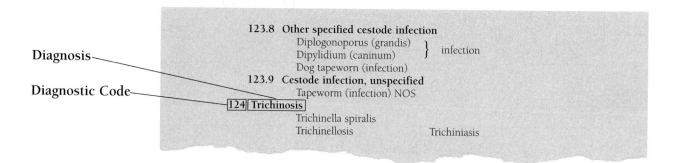

Tabular List

Figure 3-2 ICD Alphabetic Index and Tabular List

Alphabetic Index

The Alphabetic Index has three sections:

- Section 1 is the index to diseases and injuries, which are the diagnosis codes used most often. This section also contains special tables for indexing the codes for hypertension and neoplasms (tumors).
- Section 2 is a table of drugs and chemicals in alphabetic order, with corresponding codes related to poisoning and external causes.
- Section 3 is an alphabetic index of all external causes of injuries and poisonings, not just those resulting from drugs or chemicals.

The Alphabetic Index is organized by main terms in boldfaced type according to condition, as shown in Figure 3-3. A main term may be followed by a series of terms in parentheses called supplementary terms. The supplementary terms help define the main term but have no effect on the selection of the code. Because of this fact, they are referred to as "nonessential" supplementary terms. A subterm is indented underneath the main

term in regular type. Subterms do affect the selection of ap
nosis codes. They describe essential differences in body site,
cause of disease), or clinical type. Often, a main term or su
Alphabetic Index includes a cross-reference that indicates whe
for additional supplementary terms, anatomical sites, or main

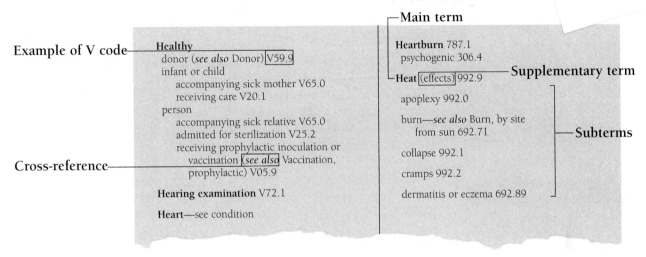

Figure 3–3 Sample of ICD Alphabetic Index with Labels

Tabular List

The Tabular List in the ICD presents diagnosis codes in numerical order.
Many illnesses are classified according to body system, so a particular group
of diseases can be found by checking the table of contents, as shown in
Table 3-1.

Table 3-1 ICD Tabular List Table of Contents

Chapter		Categories
1	Infectious and Parasitic Diseases	001–139
2	Neoplasms	140–239
3	Endocrine, Nutritional, and Metabolic Diseases and Immunity Disorders	240–279
4	Diseases of the Blood and Blood-Forming Organs	280–289
5	Mental Disorders	290–319
6	Diseases of the Central Nervous System and Sense Organs	320–389
7	Diseases of the Circulatory System	390–459
8	Diseases of the Respiratory System	460–519
9	Diseases of the Digestive System	520–579
10	Diseases of the Genitourinary System	580–629
11	Complications of Pregnancy, Childbirth, and the Puerperium	630–677
12	Diseases of the Skin and Subcutaneous Tissue	680–709
13	Diseases of the Musculoskeletal System and Connective Tissue	710–739
14	Congenital Anomalies	740–759
15	Certain Conditions Originating in the Perinatal Period	760–779
16	Symptoms, Signs, and Ill-Defined Conditions	780–799
17	Injury and Poisoning	800–999

(Table 3-1 Continued)

Supplementary Classifications

| V Codes | Supplementary Classification of Factors Influencing Health Status and Contact with Health Services | V01–V83 |
| E Codes | Supplementary Classification of External Causes of Injury and Poisoning | E800–E999 |

Appendices

A	Morphology of Neoplasms
B	Glossary of Mental Disorders
C	Classifications of Drugs by American Hospital Formulary Service List Number and Their ICD-9-CM Equivalents
D	Classification of Industrial Accidents According to Agency
E	List of Three-Digit Categories

V codes and E codes are found in numerical order following the Tabular List. V codes classify factors that influence health status or the reasons patients seek medical services when they are not ill. Examples of V codes include routine physical examinations, routine care during pregnancy, and immunizations or vaccinations.

It is appropriate to use V codes:

- When a patient is not sick but receives a service for a purpose, such as an ultrasound during pregnancy.

- When a patient with a current or recurring condition receives treatments, such as physical therapy.

- When a patient has a past condition that affects current health status or has a family history of disease.

E codes are diagnosis codes for external causes of poisonings and injuries. E codes are used *in addition to* the main code that describes the injury or poisoning itself. For example, if a person had a concussion from the impact sustained in a car accident, an E code would be used to indicate the external cause of the diagnosis. E codes are often reported on workers' compensation claims and for liability insurance, since they are used to define what happened and where it happened.

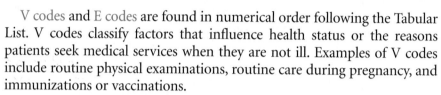

Case Study 3-3

Patient Betty Standover received an endometrial biopsy and pelvic ultrasound to monitor any changes of the endometrium that may be caused by a medication she is taking.

What type of code is used to describe the medical need for the biopsy and the ultrasound?

Answer:

V 71.83

E 881.0

V-code

Patient Frank Sherchasy fell off a ladder while on the job at Right's Painting Service. He sprained his left ankle and has a simple fracture of the right femur.

What type of code is used in addition to the main codes to describe his diagnosis?
Answer:

_____

E code

ICD-9-CM Conventions

A list of abbreviations, punctuation, symbols, typefaces, and instructional notes appears at the beginning of the ICD. These items, called conventions, provide guidelines for using the ICD system. Some key conventions are:

NOS—This abbreviation means not otherwise specified, or unspecified. This convention is used when a condition cannot be described more specifically. In general, codes with NOS should be avoided. The physician should be asked to help select a more specific code, if possible.

NEC—This abbreviation means not elsewhere classified. This convention is generally used when the ICD does not provide a code specific enough for the patient's condition. NEC should not be used as a shortcut to avoid looking up more specific codes.

[ ] Brackets—Used around synonyms, alternative wordings, or explanations.

( ) Parentheses—Used around descriptions that do not affect the code, that is, nonessential supplementary terms.

: Colon—Used in the Tabular List after an incomplete term that needs one of the terms that follow to make it assignable to a given category.

} Brace—Encloses a series of terms, each of which is modified by the statement that appears to the right of the brace.

Includes—This note indicates that the entries following it refine the content of a preceding entry. For example, after the three-digit diagnosis code for acute sinusitis, the word *includes* is followed by the types of conditions that the code covers.

Excludes—These notes, which are italicized, indicate that an entry is not classified as part of the preceding code. The note may also give the correct location of the excluded condition.

Use additional code—This note indicates that an additional code should be used, if available.

Code first underlying disease—This instruction appears when the category is not to be used as the primary diagnosis. These codes may not be used as the first code; they must always be preceded by another code for the primary diagnosis.

Diagnostic coding follows a five-step process:

Step 1—Locate the statement of the diagnosis in the patient's medical record.

Step 2—Find the diagnosis in the ICD's Alphabetic Index.

Step 3—Locate the code from the Alphabetic Index in the ICD's Tabular List.

Step 4—Read all information and subclassifications to get the code that corresponds to the patient's specific disease or condition. Note fourth- or fifth-code requirements and exclusions.

Step 5—Record the diagnosis code on the insurance claim, and proofread the numbers.

Each step is explained in the following pages. Coding becomes easier with practice, but do not be tempted to take shortcuts. Every case is different, and additional terms or digits may be necessary to make a diagnosis code as specific as possible. If a step is skipped, important information may be missed. If more than one diagnosis is listed in a patient's medical record, work on only one diagnosis at a time to avoid coding errors.

Step 1 Locate the statement of the diagnosis in the patient's medical record.

First, find the place where the physician has indicated the diagnosis. This information may be located on the encounter form or elsewhere in the patient's medical record, such as a progress note.

For example, a patient, Susan Tyne, age forty-five, comes to the office. Her medical record reads:

> CC: Chest and epigastric pain; feels like a burning inside. Occasional reflux. Abdomen soft, flat without tenderness. No bowel masses or organomegaly.
> Dx: Peptic ulcer.

Susan's diagnosis is peptic ulcer.

Then, if needed, decide which is the main term or condition of the diagnosis. For example, in Susan's diagnosis, the main term or condition is *ulcer*. The word *peptic* describes what type of ulcer it is.

Case Study 3-5

Patient: Hillary Baez
Dx: Complete paralysis.

What is the condition in this diagnosis? What is the supplementary term in this diagnosis?
Answer:

Case Study 3-6

Patient: Renate Martello
Dx: Heart palpitation.

[handwritten annotations: "supplementary", "condition" with arrows]

What is the condition in this diagnosis?
What is the supplementary term in this diagnosis?

Answer: *[crossed out handwriting]*

Case Study 3-7

Patient: Rob Blaze
Dx: Panner's disease.

[handwritten arrow]

What is the condition in this diagnosis?

Answer: *disease*

Step 2 Find the diagnosis in the ICD's Alphabetic Index.

Look for the condition first. Then find descriptive words that make the condition more specific. Read all cross-references to check all the possibilities for a term and its synonyms.

Suppose the diagnosis is sebaceous cyst. Look under *cyst,* the condition, rather than *sebaceous,* the descriptive word. Many entries in the Alphabetic Index are cross-referenced. For example, *sebaceous* is followed by instructions in parentheses that say "(*see also* Cyst, sebaceous)." Observe all cross-reference instructions.

Examine all subterms under the main term in the Alphabetic Index to be sure the correct term is found. Do not stop at the first one that "sounds right." When you find the correct term, make a note of the code that follows it.

For example, Figure 3-4 illustrates how to look up Susan Tyne's diagnosis of peptic ulcer. First, find the term *ulcer.* Notice that the term *peptic* is found in the list of subterms that follows the main term. After *peptic,* the term *(site unspecified)* appears. Since parentheses around a term indicate that it does not affect the code number, this is tentatively the correct code. (It must be verified by using the Tabular List.)

Make a note of the code, which is 533.9.

Ulcer, ulcerated, ulcerating, ulceration,
    ulcerative—*continued*

. . .

peptic (site unspecified) 533.9

Figure 3-4 Locating an Item in the Alphabetic Index

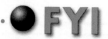
Step 3 Locate the code from the Alphabetic Index in the ICD's Tabular List.

Remember, the number to check is a code number, not a page number. The Tabular List gives codes in numerical order. Look for the number in bold-faced type. For Susan Tyne's diagnosis, look for the number 533.9 in the ICD's Tabular List.

Step 4 Read all information and subclassifications to get the code that corresponds to the patient's specific disease or condition. Note fourth- or fifth-code requirements and exclusions.

Refer to Figure 3-5, which shows all the Tabular List entries that are under the three-digit code 533. Observe all instructional notations in the list.

Next to Susan Tyne's code of 533.9, the ICD indicates "fifth code required." This note means that the correct code for the diagnosis must have five digits. In Susan Tyne's case, the diagnosis does not mention an obstruction. Therefore, the correct code is 533.90.

Notice that if this diagnosis had been peptic ulcer: duodenal or gastric, it would have been excluded from the 533 code number. The italicized word *Excludes*, boxed under the main term *Peptic ulcer, site unspecified*, is an instructional note that points to alternative code numbers.

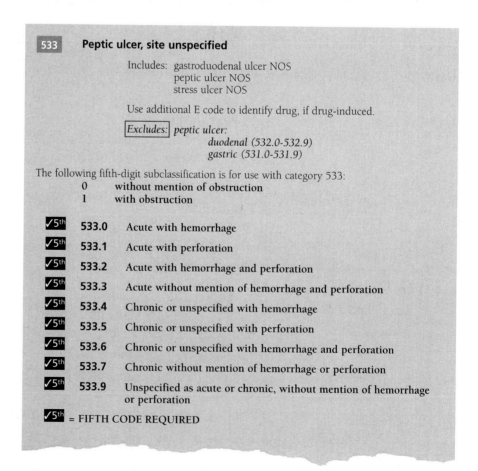

Figure 3–5 Locating an Item in the Tabular List

Step 5 Record the diagnosis code on the health care claim, and proofread the numbers on the screen.

Enter the correct diagnosis code in the medical billing program (explained in detail in Chapter 6), then proofread. The medical insurance specialist should ask these questions:

- Are the numbers entered correctly? If numbers are transposed, the insurance carrier will receive the wrong diagnosis. Proofread the numbers on the computer screen or on the printed claim form.
- Are the codes complete? If the phone rang in the middle of coding a diagnosis, the last number of the code may have been omitted.
- Is the most specific code always used?

Case Study 3-8

Using the table shown here and the following progress notes, answer the questions about this case study.

Harold Dayton's progress notes read as follows:
CC: Fatigue, chills, upset stomach, severe headache, moderate cough X 3 days, meds asa (aspirin only).
Dx: Influenza.

What is Harold Dayton's diagnosis? Use the five-step process to determine the correct ICD diagnosis code.

Answer: _Influenza 487.8_

Index to Diseases	Tabular List

Influenza, influenzal 487.1
  with
    bronchitis 487.1
    bronchopneumonia 487.0
    cold (any type) 487.1
    digestive manifestations 487.8
      hemoptysis 487.1
    involvement of
      gastrointestinal tract 487.8
        nervous system 487.8
    laryngitis 487. 1
    manifestations NEC 487.8
      respiratory 487.1
	487 Influenza
	  487.0 With pneumonia
	  487.1 With other respiratory
	    manifestations
	  ⌀ **487.8** With other manifestations

Case Study 3-9

Using the table shown here and the following progress notes, answer the questions about this case study.

Hazel Knight came to the office because of a sore, red throat. She has pus pockets in the back of her throat and has experienced fever for the past two days. A test showed streptococcal infection, Part of her examination included a blood pressure check that read 150/98. The physician diagnosed essential hypertension and streptococcal pharyngitis.

Which diagnosis is Hazel Knight's primary diagnosis?
What is the coexisting condition?
Use the five-step process to determine the correct ICD diagnosis codes.

Answer: *Streptococcal infection*

Primary code: *034.0*

Secondary code: *401.9*

Index to Diseases	Tabular List

essential—*see* condition
 	
...
 	
hypertension, hypertensive (arterial) (arteriolar)(crisis) (degeneration) (disease) (essential) ...
   malignant 401.0
   benign 401.1
   unspecified 401.9
...
pharyngitis
...
streptococcal **034.0**
	401 Essential hypertension
	   401.0 Malignant
	   401.1 Benign
	   401.9 Unspecified
	...
	
	034 Streptococcal sore throat and scarlet fever
	
	   034.0 Streptococcal sore throat
	   034.1 Scarlet fever

Case Study 3-10

Using the table shown here and the following progress notes, answer the questions about this case study.

Patient: Lee Yong
Patient is fifty-eight-year-old Asian female who presents for an annual exam.
Dx: Routine health maintenance.

What is the diagnosis?
What is the correct code?

Answer: *annual exam*

V70.0

Index to Diseases	V Codes

Health
   advice V65.4
   audit V70.0
   checkup V70.0
   education V65.4
   hazard (*see also* History of) V15.9
     specified cause NEC V15.89
   instruction V65.4
   services provided because ...
	V70 General medical examination
	   V70.0 Routine general medical examination at health care facility
	   V70.1 General psychiatric examination, requested by the authority

Using the table shown here and the following progress notes, answer the question about this case study.

Patient: Ralph Kramer

Patient reported accidental injury due to the firing of a rifle by his brother during a hunting trip.

What E code should be listed following the main diagnosis code?

Answer:

_____

E9222

Index to External Causes	E Code

Accident...
    firearm missile-*see* Shooting
 ...
 Shooting, shot E922.9
    hand gun (pistol) (revolver) E922.0...
    inflicted by other persons.
    rifle (hunting) E922.2
	E922 Accident caused by firearm missile
	 E922.0 Handgun
	 E922.1 Shotgun
	 E922.2 Hunting Rifle
	 E922.3 Military firearms

Professional Focus

Preview of ICD-10-CD

The tenth edition of the ICD was published by the World Health Organization in the mid-1990s. In the United States, the new *Clinical Modification* (ICD-10-CM) is being reviewed by health care professionals. ICD-10-CM is expected to be put into use by 2008. The major changes include:

- The ICD-10 contains 2,033 categories of diseases, 855 more than ICD-9. This creates more codes to permit more specific reporting of diseases and newly recognized conditions.
- Codes are alphanumeric, containing a letter followed by up to five numbers.
- A sixth digit is added to capture clinical details. For example, all codes that relate to pregnancy, labor, and childbirth include a digit that indicates the patient's trimester.
- Codes are added to show which side of the body is affected when a disease or condition can be involved with the right side, the left side, or bilaterally.

Although the code numbers look different, the basic systems are very much alike, and people who are familiar with the current codes will find that their training quickly applies to the new system.

Chapter Summary

1. Coding affects the payment process by giving the insurance carrier a clearly defined diagnosis that helps the carrier process the claim efficiently.

2. When a patient's medical record lists more than one diagnosis, the primary diagnosis is recorded first on the insurance claim. Additional diagnoses that occur at the same time as the primary condition and affect the patient's treatment or recovery are listed with additional diagnosis codes.

3. V codes identify encounters for reasons other than illness or injury and are used for healthy patients receiving routine services, for therapeutic encounters, for a problem that is not currently affecting the patient's condition, and for preoperative evaluations. E codes, which are never used as primary codes, classify the injuries resulting from various environmental events.

4. The ICD is divided into three volumes. ICD codes appear in lists arranged alphabetically and numerically. Medical offices use only the diagnosis codes that appear in the Tabular List (Volume 1) and the Alphabetic Index (Volume 2). ICD procedure codes (Volume 3) are used by hospitals.

5. The five steps for analyzing diagnoses and locating the correct ICD code are:

   (a) Locate the diagnosis in the patient's medical record.

   (b) Find the diagnosis in the ICD's Alphabetic Index.

   (c) Locate the code from the Alphabetic Index in the ICD's Tabular List.

   (d) Read all information and subclassifications to get the code that corresponds to the patient's specific disease or condition. Note fourth- or fifth-code requirements and exclusions.

   (e) Record the diagnosis code on the health care claim, and proofread the numbers.

Part 1. Choose the best answer.

_____ **1.** The person who determines a patient's diagnosis is the:
   a. physician
   b. medical insurance specialist
   c. nurse

_____ **2.** The person who reports the diagnosis code on the health care claim is the:
   a. physician
   b. medical insurance specialist
   c. nurse

_____ **3.** Medical insurance specialists should proofread code numbers:
   a. to ensure accuracy
   b. to perform step 3 in the five-step coding process
   c. both a and b

_____ **4.** The person who uses the procedure codes in the ICD (Volume 3) is the:
   a. medical insurance specialist in a medical office
   b. hospital coder
   c. both a and b

_____ **5.** The first step in the five-step process of diagnostic coding is:
   a. record diagnosis code on the insurance claim
   b. locate the diagnosis in the patient's encounter form or elsewhere in the medical record
   c. find the diagnosis in the ICD's Alphabetic Index

_____ **6.** The medical insurance specialist uses the five-step diagnostic coding process:
   a. until shortcuts are discovered
   b. only during training
   c. for every diagnosis

_____ **7.** Additional diagnoses that occur at the same time as the primary condition and affect its treatment or recovery are:
   a. chief complaints
   b. coexisting conditions
   c. none of the above

_____ **8.** When assigning diagnosis codes, the medical insurance specialist uses:
   a. the Alphabetic Index
   b. the Tabular List
   c. both a and b

_____ **9.** V codes are used primarily for:
   a. emergency situations
   b. medical services having no clear diagnosis or for preventive care
   c. statistical purposes in hospital reports

_____ **10.** Diagnosis codes should be proofread to be sure they are:
   a. keyed correctly
   b. complete
   c. both a and b

Part 2. Underline the main term in the following list. Then, using the Alphabetic Index and Tabular List in the most recent ICD-9-CM available to you, code the diagnostic statements.

789.0 **1.** Abdominal pain

436 **2.** Acute cerebrovascular disease

997.1 **3.** Postoperative fibrillation

780.1 **4.** Night sweats

478.5 **5.** Singer's nodule

354.0 **6.** Carpal tunnel syndrome

729.31 **7.** Popliteal fat pad hernia

133.8 **8.** Harvest itch

788.39 **9.** Urinary incontinence without sensory awareness

343.9 **10.** Little's disease, congenital

Part 3. Using the Alphabetic Index and Tabular List in the most recent ICD-9-CM available to you, code the following diagnostic statements.

611.2 **1.** Breast mass

_____ **2.** Muscle spasms

_____ **3.** Verruca plantaris

_____ **4.** Newborn vomiting

_____ **5.** Herpes zoster (NOS)

_____ **6.** Normal delivery

_____ **7.** Menopausal syndrome

_____ **8.** Diabetes, type II, uncontrolled, unspecified complication

_____ **9.** Attention deficit disorder with hyperactivity

_____ **10.** Acute pulmonary heart disease, unspecified

Part 4. **Using the most recent ICD-9-CM available to you, code the following diagnostic statements with the correct V code or E code.**

_____ **1.** Routine medical health checkup of infant at health care facility

_____ **2.** Fall from ladder

_____ **3.** Exposure to smallpox

_____ **4.** Vaccination against chickenpox

_____ **5.** Accidental poisoning from motor vehicle exhaust gas

_____ **6.** HIV positive with no HIV infection symptoms or conditions

_____ **7.** Mechanical failure of equipment during kidney dialysis

_____ **8.** Accidental poisoning by gasoline

_____ **9.** Father allergic to penicillin

_____ **10.** Exposure to HIV virus but not tested for infection

CHAPTER 4

Procedural Coding

Objectives

After completing this chapter, you will be able to define the key terms and:

1. Identify the purpose and format of the *Current Procedural Terminology* (CPT).
2. Name the three key factors (components) that influence the selection of Evaluation and Management codes.
3. Compare and contrast referral and consultation services.
4. Recognize surgical packages and laboratory panels that are coded as single procedures.
5. Describe the two types of codes in the Health Care Common Procedure Coding System (HCPCS) and discuss when they should be used.
6. Find correct procedure codes using the CPT.

Key Terms

add-on code
attending physician
Category II codes
Category III codes
Centers for Medicare and
  Medicaid Services (CMS)
code linkage *program*
consultation *second*
  approval
Current Procedural
  Terminology (CPT)

established patient
E/M code
global period
Health Care Common
  Procedure Coding System
  (HCPCS) *→material*
main number
modifier

new patient
panel
primary procedure *not thing*
procedure code
referral
surgical package
unbundle
unlisted procedures

comes up with the rules and Regulations

Why This Chapter Is Important to You

The information in this chapter will enable you to:

- Understand professional services.
- Learn to use another important reference book, the *Current Procedural Terminology*.
- Perform an essential step in the medical billing and payment process.

What Do You Think?

After making a diagnosis, the physician determines the proper course of treatment for the patient's health situation. As in diagnostic coding, the medical insurance specialist's role is to accurately communicate to the payer the procedures and services performed by the physician. Why is it important that the procedure codes relate correctly to the diagnosis?

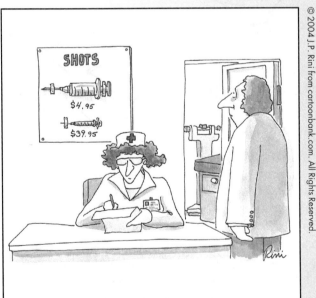

INTRODUCTION TO PROCEDURE CODES IN THE CPT

When a patient sees a physician, each procedure and service performed is reported on a health care claim using a standardized procedure code. Procedure codes represent medical procedures, such as surgery and diagnostic tests, and medical services, such as an examination to evaluate a patient's condition.

Medical insurance specialists verify procedure codes and use them to report physicians' services. The practice's physicians, medical coders, or—in some cases—medical insurance specialists are responsible for the selection of procedure codes. This chapter provides a basic introduction to procedural coding, so that you can work effectively with health care claims and encounter forms.

On correct claims, each reported service is connected to a diagnosis that supports the procedure as necessary to investigate or treat the patient's condition. Health plans analyze this connection between the diagnostic and the procedural information, called code linkage, to evaluate the medical necessity of the reported charges. Correct claims also comply with many other regulations from government agencies.

Organization of the CPT

The HIPAA-required system of procedure codes is found in the Current Procedural Terminology, published by the American Medical Association (AMA) and known as CPT. An updated edition of the CPT is published every year to reflect changes in medical practice. Newly developed procedures are added, some are changed, and old ones that have become obsolete are deleted. These changes are also available in a computer file, because some medical offices use a computer-based version of the CPT.

CPT Category I codes—which are most of the codes in CPT—are five-digit numbers, organized into six sections:

Section	Range of Codes
Evaluation and Management	Codes 99201–99499
Anesthesia	Codes 00100–01999
Surgery	Codes 10021–69990
Radiology	Codes 70010–79999
Pathology and Laboratory	Codes 80048–89356
Medicine	Codes 90281–99602

With the exception of the first section, the CPT is arranged in numerical order. Codes for evaluation and management are listed first, out of numerical order, because they are used most often. Each section opens with important guidelines that apply to its procedures. This material should be checked carefully before a procedure code is chosen.

Procedure codes are located by starting with the CPT's index, an alphabetic list of procedures, organs, and conditions in the back of the book (see Figure 4-1). Boldfaced main terms may be followed by descriptions and groups of indented terms. The correct code is selected by reviewing each description and indented term under the main term.

HIPAA Tip

New CPT codes are released around October 1 and must be used for services dated the following January 1 or later. Medical offices should have the current year's CPT available for reference because CPT codes as of the date of service—not the date of the claim preparation—are required on health care claims. Previous years' books should also be kept in case there is a question about already submitted insurance claims.

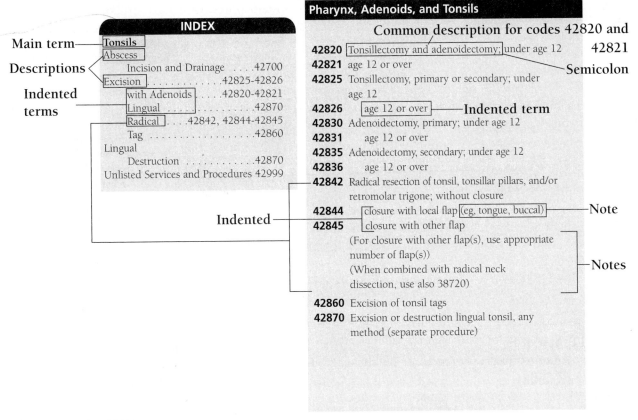

Figure 4–1 The CPT Format

The six primary sections of the CPT are divided into subsesctions. These in turn are further divided into headings according to the type of test, service, or body system. Code number ranges included on a particular page are found in the upper-right corner. This helps to locate a code quickly after using the index.

In the CPT sections, four symbols are used to highlight changes or special points. A bullet, which looks like a black circle (●), indicates a new procedure code. A triangle (▲) indicates a change in the code's description. Facing triangles (▶◀) enclose other new or revised information. A plus sign (+) is used for **add-on codes**, indicating procedures that are usually carried out in addition to other procedures. For example, code 90471 covers one immunization administration, and code 90472 covers administering an additional vaccination. Add-on codes are never reported alone. They are used together with the primary code.

The CPT uses a particular format to show codes and their descriptions. Some descriptions are indented to show that they include a common entry from above. For example, look at the descriptions for codes 42842, 42844, and 42845 in Figure 4-1. Code 42842 is the parent code in this list. Its description begins with a capital letter. Codes 42844 and 42845 are indented, and each begins with a lowercase letter. These indented codes refer to the parent code above. The words in the description of the parent code that precede the semicolon are common to all the indented codes below it. Thus, code 42844 has the full description: "Radical resection of tonsil, tonsillar pillars, and/or retromolar trigone; closure with local flap." But if the procedure is described as "closure with other flap," the correct code would be 42845.

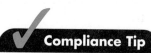
CPT listings may also contain notes, which are explanations for categories and individual codes. Notes often appear in parentheses after a code. Many times notes suggest other codes that should be considered before a final code is selected. For example, the note for code 42844 in Figure 4-1 is "(e.g., tongue, buccal)," meaning that either of these terms may appear in the description of the local flap.

One or more two-digit CPT modifiers may be assigned to a five-digit main number. Modifiers are written with a hyphen before the two-digit number. The use of a modifier shows that some special circumstance applies to the service or procedure the physician performed. For example, in the Surgery section, the modifier -62 indicates that two surgeons worked together, each performing part of a surgical procedure, during an operation. Each physician will be paid part of the amount normally reimbursed for that procedure code. Likewise, the modifier -80 indicates that the services of a surgical assistant were used, and this person's fees are a part of the claim. Appendix A of the CPT explains the proper use of each modifier. Some section guidelines also discuss the use of modifiers with the section's codes.

Unlisted Procedures, Category II Codes, and Category III Codes

Some services or procedures occur infrequently. Others are too new to be included in the CPT. Therefore, each section provides codes to be used when a service or procedure is not listed. Codes for unlisted procedures are found in the guidelines at the beginning of each section, except for Anesthesiology, where the codes are found under the Other Procedures subsection. Whenever a code for an unlisted procedure is used, a special report must be attached to the health care claim. It describes the procedure, its extent, and the reason it was performed. It also gives the equipment and amount of time and effort required.

Category II codes, listed at the end of the regular (Category I) CPT codes, are used to track performance measures for a medical goal such as reducing tobacco use. Reporting these codes on health care claims is optional, and they are not paid. They help in the development of best practice care and improve documentation. These codes have an alphabetic character for the fifth digit, such as 0002F for tobacco use, smoking, assessed.

Category III codes, also listed at the end, are temporary codes for emerging technology, services, and procedures. If a Category III code exists for a service, it must be used, rather than an unlisted code. These codes also have an alphabetic fifth digit, such as 0041T for urinalysis infectious agent detection. A temporary code may become permanent and part of the regular codes if the service it identifies proves effective and is widely performed.

CODING EVALUATION AND MANAGEMENT SERVICES

To diagnose conditions and plan treatments, physicians use a wide range of time, effort, and skill for different patients and circumstances. In the guidelines to the Evaluation and Management (E/M codes) section, the CPT

Explore the Internet

New codes are released annually on the American Medical Association Web site and published yearly in the CPT reference. Search the AMA topics on the site and read about new CPT Category II or III codes for the current year.

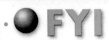

Annual physical examinations are located under the heading "Preventive medicine services" in the E/M section and are coded based on the age of new or established patients. For example, the procedure code 99395, in the established-patient category, covers the routine examination, with tests and counseling, of a patient between the ages of eighteen and thirty-nine.

explains how to choose the correct codes for different levels of these services. Three key factors documented in the patient's medical record help determine the level of service:

- The extent of the patient history taken
- The extent of the examination conducted
- The complexity of the medical decision making

In addition to level of service, health plans want to know whether the physician treated a new patient or an established patient. Physicians often spend more time during new patients' visits than during visits from established patients, so the E/M codes for the two types of patients are separate. For reporting purposes, in the CPT a new patient is one who has not received professional services from the physician within the past three years. Medical offices commonly use the abbreviation *NP* for a new patient. An established patient is one who has seen the physician within the past three years. (Note that the current visit need not be for a problem treated previously.) Medical offices commonly use the abbreviation *EP* for an established patient. Emergency patients are not classified as either new or established patients.

For example, the lowest code level for a new-patient encounter in the E/M section involves (1) a brief history, (2) an examination limited to the affected body area or organ system, and (3) a diagnostic decision made without the need for much additional information such as lab tests or X-rays. The lowest code level usually assumes a minor problem, and the time spent by the physician face-to-face with the patient is ten minutes.

Location of Service

The place where the service occurred is also important to know, because different E/M codes apply to services performed in a physician's office, a hospital inpatient room, a hospital emergency room, a nursing facility, an extended-care facility, or a patient's home.

Referrals and Consultations

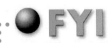

The CPT has a range of five codes each for new-patient and established-patient encounters. The lowest-level code is often called a Level I code, on up to a Level V code. For example, code 99213 is the Level III code for an established patient's office visit.

Sometimes one physician sends a patient to another physician for examination and treatment. For example, Martha Silvers is seen by Dr. House, her family practice physician. Ms. Silvers complains of shortness of breath (SOB) and recurring chest pain. Dr. House performs an electrocardiogram (ECG) and sends Ms. Silvers to Dr. Valentine, a cardiologist. Dr. House transfers Ms. Silvers's care for this condition to Dr. Valentine. This transfer is called a referral. After Dr. Valentine examines Ms. Silvers, she orders necessary tests and treatment. Since Dr. Valentine has assumed responsibility for management of Ms. Silvers's condition, the standard E/M codes for her services are used.

At other times, a physician requests advice from another physician. Suppose Dr. House asks Dr. Valentine only to perform a series of tests and report the results with an opinion to him. In this case, Dr. House remains the attending physician, the physician in charge of the patient's care. Dr. Valentine's services are coded as a consultation.

The CPT E/M section lists several codes for consultations. They differ in the level and location of service. For example, CPT code 99241 represents an office consultation involving a straightforward, relatively minor problem, such as treating a sprain. On the other hand, CPT code 99244 represents an office consultation that requires complex decision making to treat a relatively severe problem. An example is an evaluation of treatment options with a patient who has a large tumor in a breast.

Note that when a patient, not a physician, asks for a consultation with another doctor, this is called a confirmatory consultation and is coded using its own codes from the E/M section.

Professional Focus

Certification as a Medical Coder

A medical insurance specialist who wishes to study and take an examination to earn certification as a medical coder should contact one of the national accrediting associations for information. The titles of Certified Procedural Coder (CPC) and Certified Procedural Coder–Hospital (CPC-H) are granted by the American Academy of Professional Coders (AAPC), 309 West 700 South, Salt Lake City, UT 84101, Telephone: 800-626-2633, http://www.aapc.com. The American Health

Information Management Association (AHIMA) offers three coding certifications: the Certified Coding Associate (CCA), intended as a starting point for entering a new career as a coder; the Certified Coding Specialist (CCS); and the Certified Coding Specialist-Physician-based (CCS-P). American Health Information Management Association (AHIMA), 919 North Michigan Avenue, Suite 1400, Chicago, IL 60611-1683, Telephone: 312-787-2672, http://www.ahima.org.

CODING SURGICAL PROCEDURES

Codes in the Surgery section represent groups of procedures that include all routine elements. This combination of services is called a surgical package. According to the Surgery section guidelines in the CPT, the procedure codes for surgical procedures include the operation itself as well as local or topical anesthesia, one related E/M encounter to prepare the patient (immediately before or on the date of the surgery), writing orders, evaluating the patient in the recovery area, and typical follow-up care.

The procedure code for a surgical package covers a group of services that should not be listed individually. Payers assign a fee to these codes that reimburses all the services provided under them. The period of time that is covered for follow-up care is referred to as the global period. For example, the global period for repairing a tendon might be set at fifteen days. A global period for major surgery such as an appendectomy might be set at one hundred days. After the global period ends, additional services that are provided can be reported separately for additional payment.

Two types of services are not included in surgical package codes. These services are reported separately and reimbursed in addition to the surgical package fee.

- Complications or recurrences that arise after therapeutic surgical procedures.
- Care for the condition for which a diagnostic surgical procedure is performed. Routine follow-up care included in the code refers only to care related to recovery from the diagnostic procedure itself, not the condition.

When health plans pay for more than one surgical procedure performed on the same day for the same patient, they pay the full amount of the first listed surgical procedure, but they often pay less than the full amount for the other procedures. For maximum payment when multiple procedures are reported, the most complex or highest-level code—the procedure with the highest reimbursement value—should be listed first. The other procedures are listed with the modifier -51 or the modifier -59. Modifier -51 is used for multiple procedures at the same body site or system. Modifier -59 indicates distinct procedures, each fully reimbursed, rather than multiple procedures. It is usually used when the surgeon performs procedures on two different body sites or organ systems, such as the excision of a lesion on the chest as well as the incision and drainage (I & D) of an abscess on the leg.

CODING LABORATORY PROCEDURES

Organ or disease-oriented panels listed in the Pathology and Laboratory section of the CPT include tests frequently ordered together (see Figure 4-2). A comprehensive metabolic panel, for example, includes tests for albumin, bilirubin, calcium, carbon dioxide, chloride, glucose, and other factors. Each element of the panel has its own procedure code in the Pathology and Laboratory section. However, when the tests are performed together, the code for the panel must be used, rather than listing each test separately.

ORGAN/DISEASE PANEL	
Basic Metabolic Panel	80048
General Health Panel	80050
Comprehensive Metabolic Panel	80053
Obstetric Panel	80055
Lipid Panel	80061
Acute Hepatitis Panel	80074
Hepatic Function Panel	80076

Figure 4–2 Examples of Panels in the CPT

CODING IMMUNIZATIONS

Injections and infusions of immune globulins, vaccines, toxoids, and other substances require two codes, one for giving the injection and one for the particular vaccine or toxoid that is given. For example, for an influenza shot, the administration code 90471 is used for the injection, along with one of the codes for the specific vaccine, such as 90655, 90657, 90658, or 90660.

The Health Care Common Procedure Coding System, commonly referred to as HCPCS, was developed by the Centers for Medicare and Medicaid Services (CMS) for use in coding services for Medicare patients (see Chapter 9). The HCPCS (pronounced hic-picks) coding system has two levels:

- Level I codes duplicate those from the CPT.

- Level II codes are issued by CMS in the *Medicare Carriers Manual.* They are called national codes and cover many supplies, such as sterile trays, drugs, and DME (durable medical equipment). Level II codes also cover services and procedures not included in the CPT. The HCPCS codes for Level II have five characters, either numbers or letters, or a combination of both.

HCPCS modifiers, either two letters or a letter with a number, are also available for use. These modifiers are different from the CPT modifiers. For example, HCPCS modifiers may indicate social worker services or equipment rentals.

Examples of Level II codes are:

Code Number	Description
A0428	Ambulance service; basic life support, nonemergency
E0112	Crutches, underarm, wood, adjustable or fixed; pair, with pads, tips, and handgrip
J0120	Injection, tetracycline, up to 250 mg

In medical offices that use the HCPCS system, regulations issued by CMS are reviewed to determine the correct code and modifier for claims.

Explore the Internet

Study the certification opportunities for medical coders. Using your favorite search engine, visit the Web sites for the following:
- The American Health Information Management Association (AHIMA)
- The American Academy of Professional Coders (AAPC).

FIVE STEPS FOR LOCATING CORRECT CPT CODES

Five steps are used for finding procedure codes in the CPT:
Step 1—Become familiar with the CPT.
Step 2—Find the services listed on the patient's encounter form.
Step 3—Look up the procedure code(s).
Step 4—Determine appropriate modifiers.
Step 5—Record the procedure code(s) on the health care claim.

Coding procedures become easier as the coder becomes more familiar with CPT codes. In fact, most medical offices use only a limited number of procedure codes. To practice using the CPT, follow the instructions below and look up codes used in the examples to gain understanding of the format and main sections of the book.

Step 1 Become familiar with the CPT.

Read the introduction and main section guidelines and notes. For example, look at the guidelines for the Evaluation and Management section. They include definitions of key terms, such as *new and established patient, chief complaint, concurrent care,* and *counseling.* They also explain the way E/M codes should be selected.

Case Study 4-1

Study Table 1 in the guidelines for the Evaluation and Management section of the CPT.

What code range is used for emergency department services? Now turn to Appendix A. Is it correct to use modifier -21 with E/M codes? Modifier -51?

Answer: _99281-99288; yes; no_

Step 2 Find the services listed on the patient's encounter form.

The next step is to check the patient's encounter form to see which services were performed. For E/M procedures, look for clues about the extent of history, examination, and decision making that were involved. The encounter form may also indicate the amount of time the physician spent with the patient.

For example, assume that Ms. Silvers's encounter form shows an office visit for an osteoporosis evaluation. A CAT scan is performed to test bone density, so this procedure is looked up. The evaluation and management service is also coded, based on the extent of the patient's history and examination the physician performed, and the complexity of decision making.

Step 3 Look up the procedure code(s).

First, pick out a specific procedure or service, organ, or condition. Find the procedure code in CPT's index. Remember, the number in the index is the five-digit code, not a page number. For example, to find the code for dressing change, first look alphabetically in the index for the procedure. Then, turn to the procedure code in the body of the CPT to be sure the code accurately reflects the service performed. The procedure code 15852 explains the dressing change for "other than burns" and "under anesthesia (other than local)." A dressing for a burn is listed as procedure codes 16010–16030.

In some cases, the patient's medical record shows an abbreviation, synonym, or eponym (the name of a person or place for which a procedure is named). For example, the record might state "treated for bone infection." In CPT's index, the entry for Infection, Bone, is followed by the instruction "See Osteomyelitis."

Case Study 4-2

Find the correct procedure codes for the following:

Procedure: knee arthrodesis
_27580_

Organ: incision and drainage of kidney abscess
_50020_

Condition: atrial fibrillation
_33253_

To code the excision of a vaginal cyst, one might first look under Excision. There is a listing for Cyst beneath Excision, followed by a list of organs, regions, or structures involved. Look for "Vagina" to find the code. Another way to find the code is to look under Vagina and then find the listing for "Cyst Excision" beneath it.

Case Study 4-3

Find the correct procedure code for the following:

Insertion, LeVeen shunt

Answer: 49425

Although it may seem tempting to record the procedure code directly from the index, resist the shortcut. Explanations and notes in the guidelines and main sections more accurately lead to finding main numbers and modifiers that reflect the services performed. That is the only way to ensure reimbursement at the highest allowed level.

Case Study 4-4

Ms. Silvers is referred to Dr. Valentine for chest pain. The patient's encounter form on her second appointment shows a cardiovascular stress test using submaximal treadmill, with continuous electrocardiographic monitoring, with physician supervision, interpretation, and report. Find the procedure code for the procedure.

Cardiovascular stress test

Answer: 93015

(*Hint:* Look under the heading "Cardiology.")

To make the coding process more efficient, medical offices often list frequently used CPT codes on encounter forms. After seeing the patient, the physician checks off the appropriate procedures or services. An example is shown in Figure 4-3. On this example of a dermatology practice's encounter form, the E/M codes as well as common procedures are shown.

Step 4   Determine appropriate modifiers.

Check section guidelines and Appendix A to find modifiers that elaborate on details of the procedure being coded. For example, a bilateral breast reconstruction requires the modifier -50. Find the code for "breast reconstruction with free flap": 19364. To show the insurance carrier that the procedure was performed on both breasts, attach the -50: 19364-50.

Case Study 4-5

Patient Amy Wan had surgery for ingrown toenails on the great toe of each foot. Find the procedure code for the service, including any applicable modifier.

Procedure code:

11250-50

CENTRAL PRACTICE CENTER

1122 E. University Drive
Mesa, AZ 85204
602–969–4237

PATIENT NAME	APPT. DATE/TIME	
Deysenrothe, Mae J.	10/06/2008	9:30am
PATIENT NO.	**DX**	
DEYSEMA0	**1.** V70.0 Exam, Adult **2.** **3.** **4.**	

DESCRIPTION	✓	CPT	FEE	DESCRIPTION	✓	CPT	FEE
EXAMINATION				**PROCEDURES**			
New Patient				Diagnostic Anoscopy		46600	
Problem Focused		99201		ECG Complete	✓	93000	70
Expanded Problem Focused		99202		I&D, Abscess		10060	
Detailed		99203		Pap Smear		88150	
Comprehensive		99204		Removal of Cerumen		69210	
Comprehensive/Complex		99205		Removal 1 Lesion		17000	
Established Patient				Removal 2-14 Lesions		17003	
Minimum		99211		Removal 15+ Lesions		17004	
Problem Focused		99212		Rhythm ECG w/Report		93040	
Expanded Problem Focused		99213		Rhythm ECG w/Tracing		93041	
Detailed		99214		Sigmoidoscopy, diag.		45330	
Comprehensive/Complex		99215					
				LABORATORY			
PREVENTIVE VISIT				Bacteria Culture		87081	
New Patient				Fungal Culture		87101	
Age 12-17		99384		Glucose Finger Stick		82948	
Age 18-39		99385		Lipid Panel		80061	
Age 40-64	✓	99386	180	Specimen Handling		99000	
Age 65+		99387		Stool/Occult Blood		82270	
Established Patient				Tine Test		85008	
Age 12-17		99394		Tuberculin PPD		85590	
Age 18-39		99395		Urinalysis	✓	81000	17
Age 40-64		99396		Venipuncture		36415	
Age 65+		99397					
				INJECTION/IMMUN.			
CONSULTATION: OFFICE/ER				DT Immun		90702	
Requested By:				Hepatitis A Immun		90632	
Problem Focused		99241		Hepatitis B Immun		90746	
Expanded Problem Focused		99242		Influenza Immun	✓	90659	68
Detailed		99243		Pneumovax		90732	
Comprehensive		99244					
Comprehensive/Complex		99245		**TOTAL FEES**			335.00

Figure 4–3 Encounter Form with Selected Procedure Codes

Case Study 4-6

Patient Judi Goldfarb had a partial mastectomy of the left breast.

Procedure code:

_19160_

Case Study 4-7

Patient Tonisha Williams had a total abdominal hysterectomy and removal of tubes and ovaries for submucous leiomyoma of the uterus and severe polycystic disease of the ovaries.

Procedure code:

_58150_

Case Study 4-8

Established patient: Randy Kane
Visit to Ashworth Dermatology Clinic for recurrence of forearm rash. He is a previous patient who presented with this condition twenty days ago. I saw him for a ten-minute follow-up examination because of the flare-up. Has 4 × 6 cm rash over mid-forearm with scaly, erythematous, raised papules.

Procedure code:

_99212_

Case Study 4-9

Doctor LaFarge is called to the home of the BeGeorgs family. She is the family physician. The patient, thirteen-year-old son Ralph, is recovering very well from a recent urinary tract infection.

Procedure code:

_99347_

Case Study 4-10

Juanita Escobar, age two, has an intramuscular injection for immunization with diphtheria and tetanus toxoids (DT).

Procedure codes:

99392   86648

DT DPT tetanus 90702

(Hint: Check the possible codes for patients' ages.)

90471 + 90702

Step 5 Record the procedure code(s) on the health care claim.

After the procedure code is verified, it is posted to the claim. If the patient has more than one diagnosis for a single claim, the primary diagnosis is listed first (see Chapter 3). Likewise, the corresponding primary procedure is listed first. The primary procedure is the main service performed for the condition listed as the primary diagnosis.

The physician may perform additional procedures at the same time or in the same session as the primary procedure. If additional procedures are performed, match up each procedure with its corresponding diagnosis. If this is not done, the procedures will not be considered medically necessary, and the claim will be denied.

For example, Ms. Silvers, who saw Dr. House for chest pain and shortness of breath, also has asthma. While the patient is in the office, Dr. House renews her prescription for asthma medication along with performing the ECG. If the ECG is mistakenly shown as a procedure for asthma, the claim will be denied, because that procedure is not medically necessary for that diagnosis.

Chapter Summary

1. The purpose of the Current Procedural Terminology is to provide a standardized list of procedure codes for medical, surgical, and diagnostic services. It is divided into six sections: (a) Evaluation and Management, (b) Anesthesiology, (c) Surgery, (d) Radiology, (e) Pathology and Laboratory, and (f) Medicine (except anesthesiology).

2. The three main factors (components) that influence the level of service for coding purposes are the type and extent of (a) history, (b) examination, and (c) medical decision making.

3. Referral services are those performed for a patient whose care has been transferred from one physician to another. Consultation services occur when an attending physician requests advice from another physician.

4. Surgical packages and laboratory panels should be coded as single procedures rather than broken into component parts.

5. The Health Care Common Procedure Coding System (HCPCS), used to code Medicare services, has codes from CPT, as well as Level II codes.

6. To find correct procedure codes using the CPT:

   Step 1 Become familiar with the CPT.

   Step 2 Find the services listed on the patient's encounter form.

   Step 3 Look up the procedure code(s) in the Index and then cross-reference to the Main Section of the CPT code book.

   Step 4 Determine appropriate modifiers.

   Step 5 Record the procedure code(s) on the health care claim.

Check Your Understanding

Part 1. Fill in each blank with the correct answer. Then unscramble the bracketed letters to reveal a term that is a quick abbreviation for medical services.

1. The *Current Procedural Terminology* is better known as the C [P] I.

2. This section of the CPT is found at the beginning of the book, because services in it are used most often. It is called [E]VALUATIONANDMANAGEMENT.

3. A two-digit code that describes special circumstances about a procedure is called a(n) M[O]DIFIER.

4. The procedure code 23174 is found in the SEG[R]Y section of the CPT.

5. A patient who has been seen by the physician within the last three years is a(n) [E]STABLISHED patient.

6. A code that is used in addition to a primary procedure, shown in the CPT with a plus sign, is called a(n) ADD-ON[C]ODE.

7. The I N[D]EX in the back of the CPT is an alphabetic list of procedures, organs, and conditions.

8. The six sections of the CPT are Evaluation and Management, Anesthesiology, Surgery, [R]ADIOLOGY, Pathology and Laboratory, and Medicine.

9. A service performed so the physician can give advice to another physician is a(n) CONSULTATI[O]N.

10. A surgical PACKAGE is a group of related procedures and services included in the procedure code.

A quick abbreviation for a medical service is a:

ANSWER: Procedure code

Part 2. Using the most recent CPT code book available to you, find the following Evaluation and Management codes:

1. Follow-up visit, eight-year-old boy, nurse removes sutures from leg wound.

2. Office visit, twenty-nine-year-old female, established patient, follow-up on severe wrist sprain.

3. Initial office visit to evaluate gradual hearing loss, sixty-year-old female, history and physical examination, complete audiogram.

4. Initial office visit to evaluate forty-five-year-old male with complaint of shortness of breath and chest pain during exercise. Severe cardiovascular damage is suspected. Comprehensive history and examination performed. Physician spent about forty-five minutes with the patient.

5. Annual physical examination of established patient, male, age forty-two.

6. Emergency department visit for a new patient with rash over entire trunk after exposure to poison ivy.

7. Initial intensive care for E/M of critically ill baby, fifteen days old.

8. Home visit for E/M of established patient with congestive heart failure (CHF); caregiver phoned report of sudden difficulty breathing and profuse sweating.

9. Medical conference of physician and psychiatrist to discuss patient's care; approximately thirty minutes.

10. Patient, age twenty-eight, office visit for basic evaluation for life insurance.

Check Your Understanding (cont.)

Part 3. Using the most recent CPT code book available to you, find the following procedure codes:

1. Repair of nail bed.

2. Removal of twenty skin tags.

3. Radiologic examination, chest, two views, frontal and lateral.

4. Anesthesia for vaginal delivery.

5. Electrocardiogram, routine ECG, twelve leads, interpretation and report.

6. Glucose tolerance test (GTT), three specimens (includes glucose).

7. Modifier for unusual services beyond those usually required for the procedure.

8. Modifier for laboratory procedures performed by someone other than the treating or reporting physician.

9. Unlisted surgical procedure, nervous system.

10. Modifier for repeat radiology procedure performed by the same physician.

Payment Methods: Managed Care and Indemnity Plans

Objectives

After completing this chapter, you will be able to define the key terms and:

1. Discuss the major types of health plans and how the various structures affect the payments that patients owe for medical services.
2. Describe three ways in which payments to physicians are set.
3. Compare the calculation of payments for participating and nonparticipating providers, and describe how balance billing rules affect the charges that can be collected from patients.
4. List the types of charges for which a patient may be responsible at the time of a visit.

Key Terms

allowed charge
balance billing
capitation
excluded services
family deductible
fee schedule
health maintenance
  organization (HMO)
individual deductible
managed care organization
  (MCO)

nonparticipating (nonPAR)
  physician
out-of-pocket expenses
participating (PAR) physician
point-of-service (POS) plan
preferred provider
  organization (PPO)
primary care physician (PCP)
referral number

relative value scale (RVS)
Resource-Based Relative
  Value Scale (RBRVS)
usual, customary, and
  reasonable (UCR)
usual fee
walkout receipt
write off (verb)

Why This Chapter Is Important to You

The information in this chapter will enable you to:

- Become familiar with contracts between physicians and health plans and with ways of calculating physicians' payments.
- Understand the charges that are often collected from patients after office encounters.

What Do You Think?

"How much will my insurance pay?" "How much will I owe?" "Why are these doctor's fees different from my previous doctor's fees?" Questions such as these are handled by medical insurance specialists every day. What steps can the specialist take to be prepared to handle these inquiries?

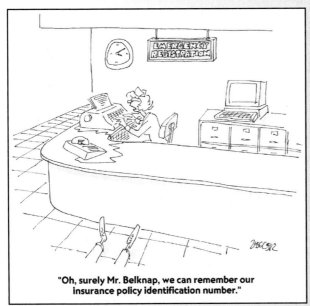

"Oh, surely Mr. Belknap, we can remember our insurance policy identification number."

Medical insurance specialists need to become familiar with the health plans that most medical offices work with. Most patients have medical coverage under one of the types of managed care plans, while some have fee-for-service plans. It is also important to learn how various types of health plans affect the way physicians are paid.

The major types of health insurance plans are summarized in Table 5-1 and described in the following section.

Table 5-1 Comparison of Major Health Plan Types

Plan Type	Provider Options	Cost Containment	Features
Preferred Provider Organization (PPO)	Network or out-of-network providers	• Referral not required for specialists • Fees are discounted • Preauthorization for some procedures	• Higher cost for out-of-network providers • Preventive care coverage varies
Health Maintenance Organization (HMO)	Network only	• Primary care physician paid by employment contract or capitation • Specialists are paid according to a contractual arrangement	• Only network provider visits covered • Covers preventive care
Point-of-Service (POS)	Network providers or out-of-network providers	• Within network, primary care physician manages care	• Lower copayments for network providers • Higher costs for out-of-network providers • Covers preventive care
Indemnity	Any provider	• Little or none • Preauthorization required for some procedures	• Higher costs • Deductibles • Coinsurance • Preventive care not usually covered

Preferred Provider Organizations

The preferred provider organization (PPO) is the leading type of managed care organization (MCO), as shown in Figure 5-1. PPOs are the most popular with patients because they combine flexibility in patients' choice of physicians with reduced cost for medical services.

A PPO is a managed care organization that creates a network of physicians, hospitals, and other health care providers for its policyholders. The providers sign contracts with the PPO under which they agree to accept reduced fees in exchange for access to a large pool of potential patients who may choose to use their services.

Patients who belong to a PPO are encouraged, but are not required, to see providers within the network. The plan pays lower benefits when services are performed by health care providers who do not belong to the PPO. For example, a larger copayment may be required when a patient sees an out-of-network provider.

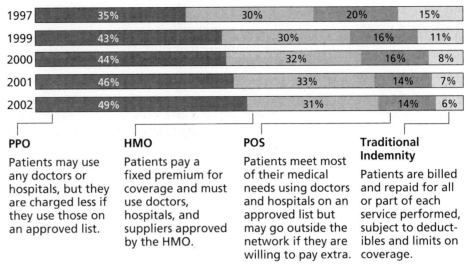

1997	35%	30%	20%	15%
1999	43%	30%	16%	11%
2000	44%	32%	16%	8%
2001	46%	33%	14%	7%
2002	49%	31%	14%	6%

PPO

Patients may use any doctors or hospitals, but they are charged less if they use those on an approved list.

HMO

Patients pay a fixed premium for coverage and must use doctors, hospitals, and suppliers approved by the HMO.

POS

Patients meet most of their medical needs using doctors and hospitals on an approved list but may go outside the network if they are willing to pay extra.

Traditional Indemnity

Patients are billed and repaid for all or part of each service performed, subject to deductibles and limits on coverage.

Source: Mercer's National Survey of Employer-Sponsored Health Plans, 2003.

Figure 5–1 Health Plan Coverage Choices in Employer-Sponsored Plans

Health Maintenance Organizations

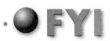

Patients should always be reminded of their financial obligations under their plans, including claim denials, according to practice procedures. The practice's financial policy regarding payment for services is usually either displayed on the wall of the reception area or included in a new patient information packet. The policy should explain what is required of the patient and when payment is due.

In health maintenance organizations (HMOs), another popular type of managed care organization, patients enroll by paying fixed premiums and very small (or no) copayments when they need services. HMOs are popular because of their low cost, although in exchange for this patients give up the flexibility of choosing their own physicians. Instead, they must use the plan's health care providers in order to have medical services covered under the plan's terms.

In some plans, a primary care physician (PCP), who is sometimes known as a gatekeeper, is assigned to each patient. This physician directs all aspects of the patient's care. The plan may require the PCP to authorize patients' visits to specialists. If so, the patient receives a referral number from the PCP that is reported to the specialist when the appointment is made.

HMOs have various contractual arrangements with providers. In some cases, physicians are employees of the HMO and work full-time seeing patients who are members of the plan. In other structures, physicians are self-employed members of the HMO's network and see both HMO policyholders and nonmember patients in their practice. In this type of structure, physicians receive a fixed payment from the HMO for each member patient, rather than reimbursement for the services provided. For each patient there is a single fee, usually paid to the PCP monthly, regardless of the number of times the patient visits the physician. This way of paying is called capitation.

Point-of-Service Plans

Because many patients do not wish to accept services from only their HMO providers, some HMOs have become point-of-service (POS) plans. Patients who choose this option do not have to use only the HMO's physicians. However, if they choose to see physicians outside the HMO's network, they must pay increased fees, such as larger copayments. This option makes the HMO more like a PPO in terms of choices available to the patients.

Indemnity Plans

Under traditional indemnity plans, the payments physicians receive are based on their regular charges for services. Currently, though, in many plans, the payer negotiates a discount for its members from the physician, just as in a PPO or POS plan. In fact, there is a great deal of overlap among the features of the various types of plans as payers attempt to control costs. Figure 5-2 provides an overview of the range of plans offered by one payer. It shows the trade-offs for patients between the lowest price and the highest flexibility. It also lists the insurance options, such as prescription drug coverage, that patients can buy from this payer.

	Maximum Provider Choice	⟵⟶		**Maximum Control of Cost and Quality**
	Indemnity	In Network or Out of Network		In Network Only
	Managed Indemnity	**PPO/Open Access**	**Point-of-Service**	**HMO/Exclusive Provider**
Network	None; use any provider	220,000 physicians 4,300 hospitals	150,000 physicians 2,000 hospitals	150,000 physicians 2,000 hospitals
Care Managed by Primary Care Physicians (PCP)	No	No	Yes: Open access OB/GYN, behavioral, vision	Yes: Open access OB/GYN, behavioral, vision
Access to Providers	May use any provider	Use any PPO network provider; may use out-of-network providers at a higher cost	Use network providers; may use out-of-network providers at a higher cost	Must use network providers
Provider Compensation	Fee-for-service, reasonable and customary rate	**In Network:** Discounted fee-for-service **Out of Network:** Fee-for-service, reasonable and customary rate	**In Network:** Capitation and discounted fee-for-service **Out of Network:** Fee-for-service, reasonable and customary rate	Capitation and discounted fee-for-service
Options	**Prescription Drug Coverage** **Behavioral Care** **Dental Care** **Vision Care** **Medicare HMO** **Life and Disability** **Expectant Mother**			

Figure 5–2 Medical Group Plans Offered by Payer

Working as a Medical Insurance Specialist

Medical insurance specialists, also called medical billers, are employed by medical group practices. They also work in clinics, for health plans, for hospitals or nursing homes, and in other health care settings. Medical insurance specialists analyze patients' medical records and collect payments for physicians' services from health plans and from patients.

Medical insurance specialists also handle the administrative work that is part of the payment process. These activities include preparing and sending insurance claims, communicating with health plans to follow up on claims, entering charges and payments in a medical billing program, and handling bill collection. They may also gather information from patients and answer written or oral questions from both patients and payers, while maintaining the confidentiality of patients' data.

Completion of a medical insurance specialist or medical assisting program at a postsecondary institution is an excellent background for an entry-level position. Professional certification, additional study, and work experience contribute to advancement to positions such as medical billing manager. Billers may also advance through specialization in a field, such as radiology billing management.

SETTING FEES

Physicians have fee schedules, lists of their fees for the procedures and services they frequently perform. These fees are called usual fees, those that they charge to most of their patients most of the time under typical conditions. Payers, too, set the fees that they pay providers. Most payers use one of three methods to set the fees that the health plan will pay physicians.

Usual, Customary, and Reasonable Payment Structure

Some health plans take the physicians' usual charges into account when they set their fee structures. The plan studies what many physicians have charged for similar services over a period of time. The fee that is set for each service is an average of the usual fee an individual physician charges for the service, the customary fee charged by most physicians in the community, and the reasonable fee for the service. This approach is called usual, customary, and reasonable (UCR).

UCR fees, for the most part, accurately reflect the charges of most physicians. However, fees may not be available for new or rare procedures. Lacking better information, a payer may set too low a fee for such procedures.

Relative Value Scale

Another method payers use to establish fees is the relative value scale (RVS) approach. Based on nationwide research, the relative value scale assigns numerical values to medical services. These values reflect the amount of skill and time the procedures require of physicians. For example, in an obstetrics practice, a hysterectomy has a higher RVS number than a dilation and curettage (D&C), because the hysterectomy is a more complicated surgical procedure and is considered to require more skill. To calculate the fee, the value assigned by the RVS is multiplied by a dollar conversion factor.

Resource-Based Relative Value Scale

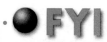

The predominant method of setting fees is based on the Centers for Medicare and Medicaid Services (CMS) Resource-Based Relative Value Scale (RBRVS). This system, which is used to set the fees for services to Medicare patients, builds on a RVS method by adding factors for the provider's expenses. Instead of valuing just the skill and time, the RBRVS also has factors for how much office overhead the procedure involves and for the relative risk that the procedure presents to the patient and to the provider (essentially the malpractice insurance expense). These factors are reflected in a mathematical formula that is used to calculate the charge for every procedure and service.

Medicare's RBRVS also takes into account the differences in costs in various areas of the United States. For example, since the cost of renting an office is higher in Chicago than in rural areas of Illinois, the compensation is different in these two locations. The RBRVS fee structure is updated every year by CMS. To calculate a particular fee, a formula taking into account the factors is multiplied by a dollar conversion factor, which is also established annually. The RBRVS method is used by many other payers. For example, one health plan may set its fees at 120 percent of the Medicare payment.

PAYMENT METHODS

After setting the fees for scheduled benefits, health plans work out various payment arrangements with providers. For example, in some cases, physicians agree to discount their usual fees. In others, physicians receive payment for each patient rather than for services.

Most payers use one of three methods of paying providers:
1. Allowed charges
2. Contracted fee schedule
3. Capitation

Payment Under an Allowed Charge Method

In the allowed charge (also called the allowable charge or maximum fee) approach, the health plan sets a payment for each covered service. The allowed charge is the maximum fee the health plan will pay for that particular service or procedure. A payer never pays a provider more than its allowed charge. If a provider's usual fee is higher, only the allowed charge is paid. If a provider's usual fee is lower, the payer pays that lower amount. The payer's payment is always the lower of the two amounts, the provider's charge or the allowable charge. For example:

The payer's allowed charge for a new patient's evaluation and management (E/M) service (CPT 99204) is $160.

Provider A Usual Charge = $180	Payment = $160
Provider B Usual Charge = $140	Payment = $140

Participating or Nonparticipating Providers

When patients have health plans that use an allowed charge payment method, physicians are paid based on whether they are participating or nonparticipating providers in that plan. A participating physician (PAR) has a contract with the managed care organization that requires accepting allowed charges—which are usually lower than the provider's usual fees—in return for incentives to be part of the plan, such as being paid faster. Nonparticipating (nonPAR) physicians have no contract with the MCO and do not agree to accept the plan's fees. Patients, of course, seek out participating physicians when they want to pay the lowest price available to them under the terms of their health plans. However, a patient may choose a nonPAR because of other factors, such as the physician's excellent reputation or advanced certification in a particular surgical procedure.

Balance Billing

The term balance billing means charging the patient for the difference between a higher usual fee and a lower allowed charge. In the example above, under balance billing, Provider A would bill the patient $20, the difference between the usual charge of $180 and the allowed charge of $160.

In most health plans that operate under allowed charge contracts, participating providers may not balance bill the patient. Instead, the PAR provider must write off the difference, meaning that the amount of the difference is subtracted from the patient's bill and never collected. A nonparticipating provider can often balance bill patients. If the nonPAR's usual charge is higher than the allowed charge, the patient must pay the difference. However, Medicare and other government-sponsored programs have different rules for nonparticipating providers, as explained in Chapters 9–12, which generally prohibit providers from balance billing patients.

Example of PAR Versus nonPAR Billing

In this example, assume that the payer's plan has an allowed charge for each procedure. The plan provides a benefit of 100 percent of the provider's usual charges, up to this maximum fee. Provider A is a participating provider; Provider B does not participate and can balance bill. Provider A and Provider B both perform abdominal hysterectomies (CPT 58150). The policy's allowed charge for this procedure is $2,880.

Provider A (PAR)
Provider's usual charge	$3,100.00
Policy pays its allowed charge	$2,880.00
Provider writes off the difference between the usual charge and the allowed charge:	$220.00

Provider B (nonPAR)
Provider's usual charge	$3,000.00
Policy pays its allowed charge	$2,880.00
Provider bills patient for the difference between the usual charge and the allowed charge ($3,000.00 – $2,880.00)	$ 120.00

There is no write-off.

Contracted Fee Schedule

Many payers, particularly PPOs and other types of managed care plans that contract directly with providers, establish fixed fee schedules with their participating providers. These payers decide what they will pay for services in particular geographical areas. Their contracts stipulate these fixed fees for the procedures and services that the plan covers. In a particular geographical area, for example, the PPO sends practices a list of fixed fees for them to consider. If the providers join the PPO network, they enter into a contract to charge patients who are enrolled in that PPO according to that fee schedule.

When a provider is working under a contracted fee schedule, the payer's allowed charge and the provider's charge are the same. The terms of the plan determine what percentage of the charges, if any, the patients owe, and what percentage the payer covers. Participating providers can typically bill patients their usual charges for procedures and services that are not covered by the plan.

Capitation

The fixed payment for each plan member in capitation contracts, called the capitation rate or cap rate, is set by the HMO that initiates contracts with providers. The plan's contract with the PCP lists the services and procedures that are covered by the cap rate. If the services are listed, the PCP must provide them for no additional charge. For example, a typical contract with a primary care provider might include the following services:

> Preventive care: well-child care, adult physical exams, gynecological exams, eye exams, and hearing exams
> Counseling and telephone calls
> Office visits
> Medical care: medical care services such as therapeutic injections and immunizations, allergy immunotherapy, electrocardiograms, and pulmonary function tests
> Local treatment of first-degree burns, application of dressings, suture removal, excision of small skin lesions, removal of foreign bodies or cerumen from external ear.

These services are covered in the per-member charge for each plan member who selects the PCP. Noncovered services can be billed to patients using the provider's usual rate. Plans often require the provider to notify the patient in advance that a service is not covered and to state the fee for which the patient will be responsible.

PATIENTS' CHARGES

Insured individuals have a variety of financial responsibilities under their health plans. Usually, a periodic premium payment is required. There are five other types of payments that patients may be obligated to pay: deductibles, copayments, coinsurance, excluded and over-limit services, and balance billing. These amounts that a patient pays are referred to as the insured's out-of-pocket expenses.

Deductibles

Most payers require policyholders to pay their deductibles before the insurance benefits begin. For example, a plan may require a patient to pay the first $200 of physician charges each year. Payments for excluded services—those that the policy does not cover—do not count toward a deductible. Some plans require an individual deductible, which must be met for each individual—whether the policyholder or a covered dependent—who has an encounter. In other cases, there is a family deductible that can be met by the combined payments to providers for any covered member(s) of the insured's family.

Copayments

Many health care plans require a patient copayment (copay). Copayments are always due and collected at the time of service. Copayments may be different for various types of services. Usually, a copay is stated as a dollar amount, such as $15 for an office visit or $10 for a prescription drug. After checking with the health plan, many offices have a policy of telling patients who are scheduling visits what copays they will owe at the time of service, so that they are prepared to pay.

Coinsurance

Many payers require coinsurance. Noncapitated health care plans such as PPOs usually require patients to pay a greater percentage of the charges of out-of-network providers than of plan providers. For example, patients may owe 20 percent of the charge when using network members but 40 percent if they go out of the network.

Excluded and Over-Limit Services

All payers require patients to pay for excluded (noncovered) services. Providers generally can charge their usual fees for these services. Likewise, in managed care plans that set limits on the annual (or other period) usage of covered services, patients are responsible for usage beyond the allowed number. For example, if one preventive physical examination is permitted annually, additional preventive examinations are paid for by the patient. Figure 5-3 shows an example of an agreement used by medical offices to notify patients of the expected fees for excluded services.

Sample Agreement for Patient Payment of Excluded Services

Service to be performed: _____

Estimated charge: _____

Date of planned service: _____

Reason for exclusion: _____

I, _____, a patient of _____, understand the service described above is excluded from my health insurance. I am responsible for payment in full of the charges for this service.

Figure 5–3 Sample Agreement for Patient Payment of Excluded Services

Balance Billing

Patients may be responsible for the amount of the usual charge that exceeds the payer's allowed charge.

Charges Due at Time of Service Versus Charges Billed

Explore the Internet

Insurance companies provide valuable information on their Web sites, such as coverage bulletins, available plans, and benefits. Visit the Web site of a major carrier, and explore its health plan information. Two suggestions are CIGNA and AETNA.

When a patient has an encounter with a participating provider, the provider files the health care claim, receives payments directly from the payer, and agrees to accept the payer's allowed charge. Patients are billed for charges that payers deny or do not pay. The following types of patient charges, however, are customarily collected at the time of service:

- Copayments
- Usual fees for services that are excluded under the patient's plan
- Usual fees for services to patients performed by nonparticipating providers (except for government-sponsored programs) and HMO out-of-network providers

When a patient has an encounter with a nonparticipating (nonPAR) provider, the procedure is usually different. To avoid the difficulty of collecting patient payments at a later date, a practice may either (1) require the patient to assign benefits, so that the physician receives the payment, or (2) require payment in full at the time of service.

If the provider has not accepted assignment and is not going to file a claim for a patient, the medical billing program is used to create a walkout receipt for the patient. The walkout receipt summarizes the services and charges for that day, as well as any payment the patient made (see Figure 5-4).

Patients may use the walkout receipt to report the charges and the payments they made to the insurance company. In this case, the insurance company repays the patient (or insured) after the deductible is met, according to the terms of the plan. In other cases, the medical office collects payment from the patient and then sends a claim to the insurance company for the patient. The insurance company sends a check to the patient with an explanation of benefits, with a copy to the provider. In still other cases, patients arrange to be billed for payments due. In this case, the billing program issues an invoice when the practice's bills are generated (see Chapter 7).

Estimating Patients' Charges

Many times, patients want to know what their bills will be. To estimate charges, the medical insurance specialist contacts the patient's health plan and verifies:

- The patient's deductible amount and whether it has been paid in full, the covered benefits, and coinsurance or other patient financial obligations
- The payer's allowed charges or the contracted fees for the services that the provider anticipates providing

If the patient's request comes after the encounter, the medical insurance specialist can use the encounter form to tell the payer what CPT codes are going to be reported on the patient's claim to learn the likely payer reimbursement.

CENTRAL PRACTICE CENTER
1122 E. University Drive
Mesa, AZ 85204
602–969–4237

Page: 1   10/1/2008

Patient: Walter Williams
17 Mill Rd
Chandler, AZ 85246-4567

Instructions:
Complete the patient information portion of your insurance
claim form. Attach this bill, signed and dated, and all other
bills pertaining to the claim. If you have a deductible policy,
hold your claim forms until you have met your deductible.
Mail directly to your insurance carrier.

Chart #: WILLIWA0
Case #: 8

Date	Description	Procedure	Modify	Dx 1	Dx 2	Dx 3	Dx 4	Units	Charge
10/1/2008	EP Problem Focused	99212		401.1	780.7			1	46.00
10/1/2008	ECG Complete	93000		401.1	780.7			1	70.00
10/1/2008	Aetna Copayment Charge	AETCOPAY		401.1	780.7			1	15.00
10/1/2008	Aetna Copayment	AETCOPAY						1	-15.00

Provider Information

Provider Name:	Christopher Connolly M.D.
License:	37C4629
Commercial PIN:	
SSN or EIN:	16-1234567

Total Charges:	$ 131.00
Total Payments:	-$ 15.00
Total Adjustments:	$ 0.00
Total Due This Visit:	**$ 116.00**
Total Account Balance:	$ 116.00

Assign and Release: I hereby authorize payment of medical benefits to this physician for the services described
above. I also authorize the release of any information necessary to process this claim.

Patient Signature: _____   Date: _____

Figure 5–4 Sample Walkout Receipt

Chapter Summary

1. The leading type of health plan, the preferred provider organization (PPO), creates a network of providers for its policyholders. Patients pay premiums and copayments, and may have deductibles to satisfy. PPOs pay lower benefits, such as requiring a larger copayment, when patients receive services from providers who do not belong to the network. Patients in a health maintenance organization (HMO) pay low fees, usually a premium and a copayment, but must use the services of HMO providers to be covered. Patients in point-of-service (POS) plans have options to see providers outside of the network for higher fees. Fee-for-service (indemnity) plan holders pay annual premiums, deductibles, and coinsurance for visits.

2. Payments to physicians are based on the usual, customary, and reasonable (UCR) method; the relative value scale (RVS) method; or the resource-based relative value scale (RBRVS) method.

3. Payers pay participating providers according to the allowed charge, contracted fee schedule, or cap rate in their contracts with the health plan. Nonparticipating physicians are usually paid according to their usual fees. If balance billing is allowed, the physician may collect the difference between a higher usual fee and the lower fee the health plan pays. Usually, only nonparticipating physicians can balance bill private-plan patients; government programs often prohibit this activity.

4. Patients may be responsible for copayments, excluded services, over-limit usage, and coinsurance. Patients often must also meet deductibles before receiving benefits. Under some conditions, patients may also be obligated to pay the difference between a provider's higher usual fee and a payer's lower allowed charge.

Check Your Understanding

Part 1. Choose the best answer.

_____ **1.** The only type of managed care organization that employs physicians directly is:
   a. a health maintenance organization (HMO)
   b. a preferred provider organization (PPO)
   c. a physician-hospital organization (PHO)

_____ **2.** In an HMO, the primary care physician is:
   a. the first physician who recommends surgery for a patient who later gets a second opinion
   b. the first physician to diagnose a patient's illness
   c. the physician who supervises all aspects of a patient's health care

_____ **3.** A physician who is a participant in a program must write off:
   a. deductibles
   b. denied or excluded charges
   c. charges in excess of the allowed amount

_____ **4.** The method that Medicare uses to establish allowed charges is:
   a. UCR
   b. RBRVS
   c. capitation

_____ **5.** The fee for a service that is charged by a provider for most patients is called the:
   a. cap rate
   b. usual fee
   c. write off

_____ **6.** Balance billing means to bill the patient for the difference between the:
   a. cap rate and the allowed amount
   b. UCR fee and the usual fee
   c. allowed amount and the usual fee

_____ **7.** The amount that an insured person must pay annually before receiving benefits from the health plan is called the:
   a. deductible
   b. cap rate
   c. allowed charge

_____ **8.** If a participating physician's usual fee is $400 and the allowed amount is $350, what amount is written off?
   a. zero
   b. $50
   c. $75

_____ **9.** The RBRVS fee-calculation method for a procedure takes into account:
   a. the time and skill of the physician
   b. regional cost differences
   c. both a and b

_____ **10.** A point-of-service option in an HMO plan allows patients:
   a. to see doctors not in the plan for an additional cost
   b. to visit doctors anywhere in the United States
   c. to select their own specialists at no additional cost

Part 2. Based on the following information, answer the questions in each case.

1. A patient's insurance policy states:

   Annual deductible: $300.00

   Coinsurance: 70-30 *30%*

   This year, the patient has made payments totaling $533.00 to all providers. Today, the patient has an office visit (fee: $80.00). The patient presents a credit card for payment of today's bill. What is the amount that the patient should pay? *$24*

2. A patient is a member of a health plan with a 15 percent discount from the provider's usual fees and a $10.00 copay. The days' charges are $480.00. What are the amounts that the plan and the patient each pay?

3. A patient is a member of a health plan that has a 20 percent discount from the provider and a 15 percent copay. If the day's charges are $210.00, what are the amounts that the plan and the patient each pay?

$80 $5 3
$72
+ ÷ 2)3.0
$10 15%
210.00
.15

CHAPTER 6
Health Care Claim Preparation and Transmission

Objectives

After completing this chapter, you will be able to define the key terms and:

1. Describe the process of using medical billing programs to prepare health care claims.
2. Briefly describe the information contained in the five major sections of the HIPAA claim.
3. Discuss the importance and use of claim control numbers and line item control numbers.
4. Identify the three major methods of electronic claim transmission.

Key Terms

audit-edit claim response
billing provider
birthday rule
claim attachment
claim control number
CMS-1500 claim form
coordination of benefits (COB)
database
data element
destination payer
edit

electronic data interchange (EDI)
HIPAA claim
HIPAA Electronic Health Care Transaction and Code Sets (TCS)
HIPAA Security Rule
line item control number
National Patient ID
National Payer ID
National Provider Identifier (NPI)

password
pay-to provider
place of service (POS) code
primary insurance
secondary insurance
referring physician
rendering provider
subscriber
taxonomy code
transactions
verification report

Why This Chapter Is Important to You

The information in this chapter will enable you to:

- Understand the information that is needed to prepare complete, accurate health care claims.
- Gain practice with case studies similar to situations you will encounter in a medical office.
- Learn the methods used to transmit correct health care claims.

What Do You Think?

To complete health care claims, medical insurance specialists work constantly with numbers—billing software, Web sites, diagnosis codes, procedure codes, fees and charges, identification numbers, preauthorization numbers, and more. Why is it important to know how to use available resources in the medical office to research or verify information? What role do accurate data entry and proofreading have in this process?

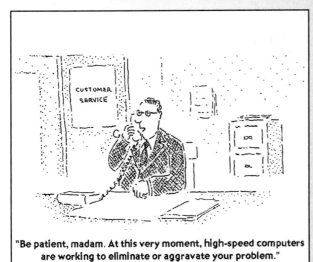

"Be patient, madam. At this very moment, high-speed computers are working to eliminate or aggravate your problem."

When preparing claims, medical insurance specialists work with computerized billing programs, following these steps:

- Record patients' information and determine the primary insurance plan
- Record services, charges, and payments for patients' encounters
- Create and transmit claims to payers

Recording Patients' Information

The first step in preparing claims is recording patients' information from new or updated patient information forms. A new record must be created for a new patient, and facts about established patients may need to be updated. Some medical offices handle this step before the patient's visit as part of the patient scheduling and registration process. Others enter the data in the medical billing program after the patient's encounter and the subsequent documentation of the patient's chief complaint, diagnosis, and expected course of treatment.

Primary Plan

Some patients have more than one insurance policy. A patient may have coverage under more than one group plan, such as a person who has both employer-sponsored insurance and a policy from union membership. In order to know which payer to bill first, the medical insurance specialist must determine which plan is primary. A person may have primary insurance coverage from an employer, but also be covered as a dependent under a spouse's insurance, making the spouse's plan the person's secondary insurance.

A common issue involves determining which of two parents' plans is primary for a child. If both parents cover dependents on their plans, the child's primary insurance is usually determined by the birthday rule. This rule states that the parent whose day of birth is earlier in the calendar year is primary. For example, Rachel Foster's mother and father both work and have employer-sponsored insurance policies. Her father, George Foster, was born on October 7, 1971, and her mother, Myrna, was born on May 15, 1972. Since the mother's date of birth is earlier in the calendar year (although the father is older), her plan is Rachel's primary insurance. The father's plan is secondary for Rachel.

Coordination of Benefits

Table 6-1 summarizes the facts that are used to determine which plan is primary. Determining the primary policy is important because under state and/or federal law, insurance policies contain a provision called coordination of benefits (COB). The coordination of benefits guidelines ensure that when a patient is covered under more than one policy, maximum appropriate benefits are paid, but without duplication. If the patient has signed an assignment of benefits statement, it is the provider's responsibility to supply the information about the secondary insurance coverage to the primary payer. This information is included in the claim to the primary payer. When the RA is received, the medical insurance specialist prepares another claim for the secondary payer, which reports the amount the first insurance policy paid and the patient's balance. After both carriers have made payments, any unpaid bills are submitted to the patient.

Table 6-1 Determining Primary Coverage

- If the patient has only one policy, it is primary.
- If the patient has coverage under two plans, the plan that has been in effect for the patient for the longest period of time is primary. However, if an active employee has a plan with the present employer and is still covered by a former employer's plan as a retiree or a laid-off employee, the current employer's plan is primary.
- If the patient is also covered as a dependent under another insurance policy, the patient's plan is primary.
- If an employed patient has coverage under the employer's plan and additional coverage under a government-sponsored plan, such as Medicare, the employer's plan is primary.
- If a retired patient is covered by a spouse's employer's plan, and the spouse is still employed, the spouse's plan is primary, even if the retired person has Medicare.
- If the patient is a dependent child covered by both parents' plans, and the parents are not separated or divorced (or if the parents have joint custody of the child), the primary plan is determined by the birthday rule.
- If two or more plans cover dependent children of separated or divorced parents who do not have joint custody of their children, the children's primary plan is determined in this order:
  —The plan of the custodial parent
  —The plan of the spouse of the custodial parent (if the parent has remarried)
  —The plan of the parent without custody

Recording Services, Charges, and Payments for Patients' Encounters

After the patient's visit with the medical professional staff, the diagnosis codes and the procedure codes are recorded in the billing program. The provider the patient saw is selected from the billing program's list of the practice's physicians and other staff. The appropriate transactions for the visit are also entered. Transactions include all the financial aspects of the visit—the charges and any payments the patient has made, such as a copayment. The source of the codes, charges, and payment information is the encounter form. The patient's appropriate insurance coverage for this visit is also selected. Usually, it is the patient's main health plan, but if the case is for a workers' compensation claim, that insurance is selected.

Creating and Transmitting Claims to Payers

When all required data elements—patient information and transactions—have been entered and checked, the medical insurance specialist instructs the billing program to create a claim for the appropriate payer. Following its programmed instructions, the program draws the needed facts from the stored information and organizes these data elements into an electronic claim file. Claims generated by billing programs can be transmitted as electronic claims to payers, or printed and mailed to them. Most health care claims are submitted electronically, not on paper.

ACCURACY AND SECURITY ISSUES

Medical billing programs increase efficiency because repeatedly used data are stored in databases—collections of related facts—and quickly accessed. For example, the office's frequently used diagnosis and procedure codes, as well as fee schedules, are entered once and then stored. A medical insurance specialist who is posting (that is, entering) the information from the encounter form does not have to enter a complete code and its description. That information has already been stored, so the correct code can be chosen from a list on the screen.

The major databases in billing programs are:

- Provider—The provider database has information about the physician(s) as well as the medical office, such as the practice's name, address, phone number, and medical identifier numbers.

- Patient/Guarantor—The data from each patient information form are stored in the patient/guarantor database. These data include the patient's unique chart number and personal information: name, address, phone number, birth date, Social Security number, gender, marital status, employer, and guarantor (the insured person if other than the patient).

- Insurance Carriers—The insurance carrier database contains the names, addresses, plan types, and other data about the major health plans used by the practice's patients.

- Diagnosis Codes—The diagnosis code database contains the ICD-9-CM codes that indicate the reason a service is provided. The codes stored are those most frequently used by the office. Additional codes can easily be entered.

- Procedure Codes—The procedure code database contains the data needed to create charges. The CPT codes most often used by the office are selected for this database. Like the ICD codes, additional CPT codes are easy to enter if needed. Other claim data, such as place of service (POS) codes and the charge for each procedure, are stored in this database.

- Transactions—The transaction database stores information about each patient's visit charges and the related diagnoses and procedures, as well as received and outstanding payments.

Data Entry

Although medical billing programs increase efficiency and reduce errors, they are not more accurate than the individual who is entering the data. If humans make mistakes while entering data, the information the computer produces will be incorrect. Computers are very precise and also very unforgiving. While the human brain knows that *flu* is short for *influenza*, the computer regards them as two distinct conditions. If a computer user accidentally enters a name as *ORourke* instead of *O'Rourke*, a human might know what is meant; the computer does not. It would probably respond with a message such as "No such patient exists in the database."

Many human errors occur during data entry, such as pressing the wrong key on the keyboard. Other errors are a result of a lack of computer literacy—not knowing how to use a program to accomplish tasks. For this reason, having proper training in data-entry techniques, so that errors are caught, and knowing how to use computer programs are both essential for medical insurance specialists. Follow these tips for accurate data entry when entering data in medical billing programs:

- Do not use prefixes for people's names, such as Mr., Ms., or Dr.
- Unless required by a particular insurance carrier, do not use special characters such as hyphens, commas, or apostrophes.
- Use only valid data in all fields; avoid words such as *same*.
- Enter the required number of characters for each data element, such as four numbers for the year, but do not worry about the format; most billing programs or claim transmission programs automatically reformat data such as dates correctly.

Data Security

The HIPAA Security Rule, another part of HIPAA regulations, sets standards for protecting individually identifiable health information (PHI) when it is maintained or transmitted electronically. Any information that is stored in a computer is being maintained electronically, so a number of security measures are often used in medical offices to enforce the HIPAA Security Rule.

- Access Control and Passwords—Most medical offices restrict access to PHI to those who need the information. Employees are given user IDs and passwords that permit using the files to which they have been granted access rights. For example, a biller needs access to patients' insurance information and medical codes and charges, but not to the medical record that documents conditions. The password would allow access to just the needed files in the electronic health record.
- Backups—Backing up is the practice of copying files to another medium so that they will be preserved in case the originals are no longer available. In medical offices, regular backups are made in case there is a security incident that jeopardizes critical data.
- Security Policy—Medical offices have a security policy, including being sure that employees are informed about their own responsibilities for protecting electronically stored information.

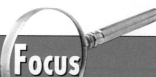

Professional Focus

Billing Services

A billing service is a company that provides data entry and claims processing services to providers for a fee. Many small practices do not have the time, knowledge, or staff available to create and process claims in-house. Some large practices may decide, too, that they would rather not develop the expertise necessary for health care claim preparation and transmission. A billing service offers a viable alternative. The medical office gives the billing service the information it needs to create claims, including patient information forms, insurance cards, and encounter forms. The billing service staff inputs the data, creates claims, and submits claims either directly to payers or to a clearinghouse, which performs an edit and then submits the claims in HIPAA format.

TYPES OF CLAIMS

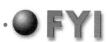

Two types of claims, HIPAA and paper, are in use. The HIPAA claim is an electronic transaction that is also called the 837 claim, for its formal name. The paper format is known as the CMS-1500 claim form (formerly the HCFA-1500).

The HIPAA claim follows the requirements of the HIPAA Electronic Health Care Transaction and Code Sets (TCS) standards. Like the HIPAA Privacy Rule and Security Rule, the HIPAA Electronic Health Care Transaction and Code Sets standards is a national regulation for all providers and payers in the health care industry. For example, the data elements for diagnoses must be ICD-9-CM codes, rather than medical terminology or codes from any other system.

The most important differences between HIPAA claims and paper claims are that:

- HIPAA claims can contain much more information than paper claims, so fewer questions and answers have to be exchanged between the medical office and the payer after the claim is sent.
- HIPAA claims must be sent as electronic files following a certain format.
- HIPAA claims must be accepted by all payers. Payers also cannot ask for their own forms or any data in place of HIPAA-standard data.

HIPAA claims are required by the Centers for Medicare and Medicaid Services (CMS) for reporting Medicare services. Only very small practices and those that never send any electronic health care transactions are exempt from this requirement. Some private payers may accept paper claims as well as HIPAA claims. However, it is anticipated that, for cost reasons, all payers will eventually require HIPAA claims and add this provision to their contracts with providers.

Since medical insurance specialists handle mostly HIPAA claims, this chapter covers the essential information that these claims require and discusses how a HIPAA claim is sent to a payer. Basic instructions for completing the CMS-1500 are also included.

The HIPAA claim has five major sections:
1. Provider information
2. Subscriber (guarantor/insured/policyholder) and patient (the subscriber or another person) information
3. Payer information
4. Claim details
5. Services

Provider Information

Information in the first section of the claim covers the provider. The billing provider is the organization or person transmitting the claim to the payer. The pay-to provider is the organization or person that should receive payment (see Figure 6-1). This distinction is necessary because medical offices often hire other firms, such as a billing service or a clearinghouse, to send their claims to payers. When this is done, the outside organization is the billing provider, and the medical practice is the pay-to provider that will receive payment from the health plan. A practice that sends claims directly to the payer is both the billing provider and the pay-to provider for those claims, so there is no additional pay-to provider to report.

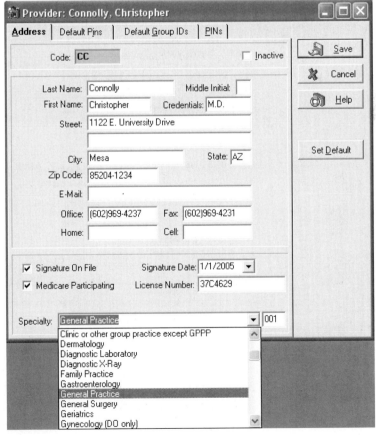

Figure 6-1 Example of Billing Program Screen for Taxonomy Code Selection   *Courtesy NDCMedisoft*

National Provider Identifier

Provider information includes the name, address, and National Provider Identifier (NPI), a ten-digit number. Another provider identifier number—such as a state license number—may also be required by some payers for their participating physicians.

Taxonomy Code

Another type of code that may be reported is a taxonomy code, a ten-digit number that stands for a physician's medical specialty. An example is 207NP0225X for pediatric dermatology. Many medical billing programs store a taxonomy code database (see the list of medical specialties in Figure 6-1). The biller selects a specialty, and the code is properly stored for the claim.

A taxonomy is reported when the type of specialty affects the physician's pay because of the payer's contractual terms. For example, nuclear medicine is a higher-paid specialty than internal medicine. An internist who is also certified in nuclear medicine would report the nuclear medicine taxonomy code when billing for a related service and use the internal medicine taxonomy code on internal medicine claims.

Subscriber/Patient Information

A second section of data elements describes the subscriber, who is the insurance policyholder or guarantor (Figure 6-2). The subscriber may be the patient, but if the subscriber and patient are not the same person, data elements about the patient are also required.

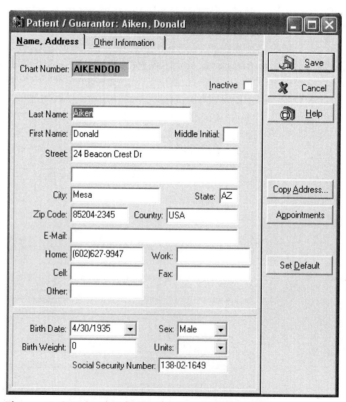

Figure 6–2 Example of Billing Program Screen for Patient Information   *Courtesy NDCMedisoft*

Explore the Internet

Visit the Web site of the National Uniform Claim Committee (NUCC) to locate information on taxonomy codes: http://www.nucc.org

HIPAA Tip

Under HIPAA, the Department of Health and Human Services (HHS) must adopt a standard system for a **National Patient ID,** an individual identifier that will be assigned to each patient in the United States who receives treatment. When this system is in place, the National Patient ID will be used instead of the health plan member number. A standard health plan identifier system must also be adopted. Each plan's number will be its **National Payer ID.** This will take the place of claim filing indicator codes.

The subscriber's complete name and health plan member number are provided. The name and number must exactly match the way they appear on the insurance card. The insured's group or policy number, group or plan name, and a claim filing indicator code are also reported. The claim filing indicator code shows the type of health plan for the claim, such as a code 12 for a PPO. These codes, which are shown in Table 6-2, are to be used until a National Payer ID system is created, as HIPAA requires.

Table 6-2 Common Claim Filing Indicator Codes

Code	Definition
09	Self-pay
12	Preferred provider organization (PPO)
13	Point-of-service (POS) plan
15	Indemnity insurance
BL	Blue Cross and Blue Shield
CH	CHAMPUS (TRICARE)
CI	Commercial insurance company
DS	Disability
HM	Health maintenance organization
MB	Medicare Part BM
MC	Medicaid
WC	Workers' compensation health claim

Relationship of Patient to Subscriber

If the subscriber is the patient, the billing program enters the correct code when the biller chooses self to describe the relationship of the patient to the subscriber. When the patient and the subscriber are not the same person, the relationship must be selected, and the medical billing program stores the right code. The HIPAA choices are shown in Table 6-3. Note that many billing programs used to limit the options to self, spouse, child, and other; these programs must be updated for HIPAA requirements so that the particular relationship can be correctly reported. This information is important, because it may affect the payment under the policy's particular statement of benefits.

Table 6-3 Relationships

Adopted child	Injured plaintiff
Child	Life partner
Child where insured has no financial responsibility	Mother
	Nephew or niece
Dependent of a minor dependent	Other adult
Emancipated minor	Other relationship
Employee	Significant other
Father	Sponsored dependent
Foster child	Stepson or stepdaughter
Grandson or granddaughter	Unknown
Handicapped dependent	Ward

Patient Information

Patient information includes the complete name, address (or "unknown," if not available for reporting), gender, date of birth, and a primary identifier, such as a health plan member ID. (The National Patient ID will be required when it is mandated for use.) Secondary identifiers, such as a Social Security number, may also be required by some payers.

Payer Information

The payer information section contains data elements about the payer to which the claim is going to be sent, called the destination payer (Figure 6-3). The payer's name and ID are required data elements (the National Payer ID will be used when legislated). An assignment-of-benefits code indicates whether the insured authorizes benefits to be paid to the provider. A referral number or prior authorization number that the payer assigned is required when a referral or preauthorization was obtained.

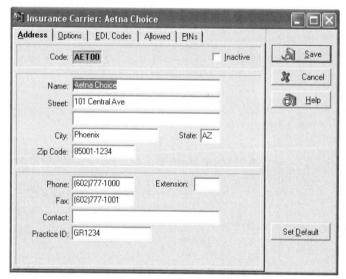

Figure 6–3 Example of Billing Program Screen for Payer Information   *Courtesy NDCMedisoft*

Claim Information

The claim information section reports information related to the particular claim. For example, if the patient's visit is the result of an accident, this fact is reported in the claim information section. Data elements about the rendering provider—the medical professional who performed the service—are provided if this was not the same as the billing provider or the pay-to provider. If another provider referred the patient for care, the claim has the name and NPI (and sometimes the taxonomy code) of the referring physician or primary care physician (PCP).

Claim Control Number

A unique claim control number is assigned by the medical insurance specialist (the sender) to each claim. The maximum number of characters is twenty. Like a return address on an envelope, the claim control number will appear on payments that come back from payers (see Chapter 7), so it is very important for tracking purposes. The claim control number should not be the same as the medical office's account number for the patient. It is a different, unique number for each claim sent for that patient. It may, however, incorporate the account number. For example, if the account number is A1234, a three-digit number might be added for each claim, beginning with A1234001.

Total Charges

The total submitted charges are entered. If the patient made any payment for the claim, this dollar amount is also entered.

Place of Service Code

The place of service (POS) code, also called the facility type code, identifies where the services reported on the claim were performed. Table 6-4 shows typical codes for physician practice claims. This code is important because payers may authorize different payments for different locations.

Table 6-4 Selected Place of Service Codes

Code	Definition	Code	Definition
11	Office	23	Emergency room—hospital
12	Home	24	Ambulatory surgical center
21	Inpatient hospital	31	Skilled nursing facility
22	Outpatient hospital	81	Independent laboratory

Diagnosis Codes

Up to eight diagnosis codes from the ICD-9-CM are reported, in any order (Figure 6-4). Each diagnosis code must be directly related to the patient's treatment. Up to four of these codes can be linked to each procedure code that is reported in the next section, service line information. Note that the decimal point in the ICD-9-CM code is not entered in electronic billing.

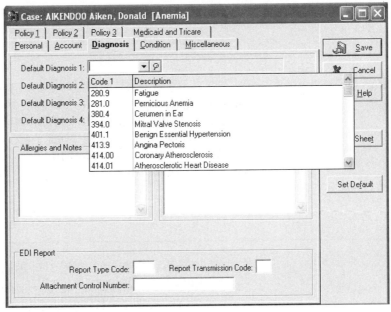

Figure 6–4 Example of Billing Program Screen for Claim Information
Courtesy NDCMedisoft

Service Line Information

The service line information section lists the procedures—that is, the services—performed for the patient (see Figure 6-5). Each service line is assigned a line item control number. Like the claim control number, these numbers are used to track payments from the insurance carrier, but for a particular service rather than the entire claim.

Each service line also has a procedure code (with a modifier, if appropriate), a date, and a charge. Also, up to four diagnosis codes can be linked to each service line procedure. At least one diagnosis code is required; codes two, three, and four may also be linked.

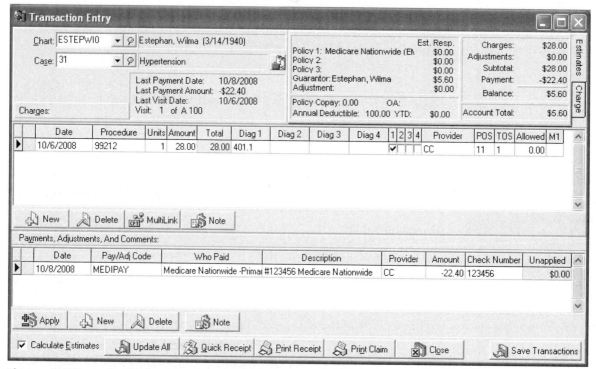

Figure 6–5 Example of Billing Program Screen for Service Line Information   *Courtesy NDCMedisoft*

Claim Attachments

A claim attachment is an additional printed form or electronic record needed to process a claim. A HIPAA transaction standard for electronic health care claim attachments is under development. Until a standard is mandated, health plans have the right to require providers to submit claim attachments in the format they specify. Attachments that are sent separately from the main claim file may be paper or electronically based.

TRANSMITTING HIPAA CLAIMS

HIPAA Tip

The verification report should be printed and filed.

Before the batch of claims is sent, the medical insurance specialist checks a verification report. This report lists the claims that are ready to be sent and includes key information for each claim. An example of a verification report is shown in Figure 6-6. It provides an opportunity to double-check that the intended batch of claims is complete and correct.

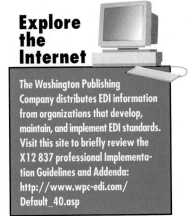
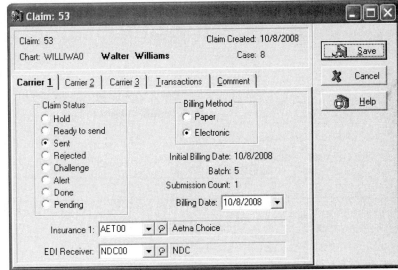

Figure 6–6 Example of Billing Program Claim Verification Report
Courtesy NDCMedisoft

Electronic Data Interchange

Transmitting HIPAA claims involves electronic data interchange, or EDI. EDI is the computer-to-computer exchange of routine business information using publicly available standards. HIPAA requires a particular EDI format, called the X12, for transmission. It also requires that, when claims are sent, patients' protected health information (PHI) must remain secure and private.

Methods of Sending Claims

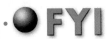

Claims are prepared for transmission after the data elements have been entered and checked. The billing program claim screen, such as that seen in Figure 6-7 on page 104, is used to monitor the transmission process. There are three major methods of transmitting claims electronically: clearinghouses, direct transmission, and direct data entry (DDE).

Clearinghouses

Most providers pay clearinghouses to receive their claims and put them in the correct EDI format for HIPAA-standard transmission. Clearinghouses must receive all required data elements because they are prohibited by HIPAA from creating or modifying data content.

Clearinghouses perform edits on claims before sending them on to payers. An edit is a computer check for missing data, such as the birth date of a patient, or mistakes, like outdated codes. An audit/edit claim response is returned electronically by the clearinghouse to the provider. It lists the problems that would cause the claim to be rejected by the payer and asks the sender to correct the errors. When this has been done and all claim information is resent correctly, the clearinghouse transmits the clean claim to the appropriate payer. (Claims with missing information or that fail other edit screens, such as use of a gender-specific procedure code for a patient of the wrong sex, are called dirty claims.)

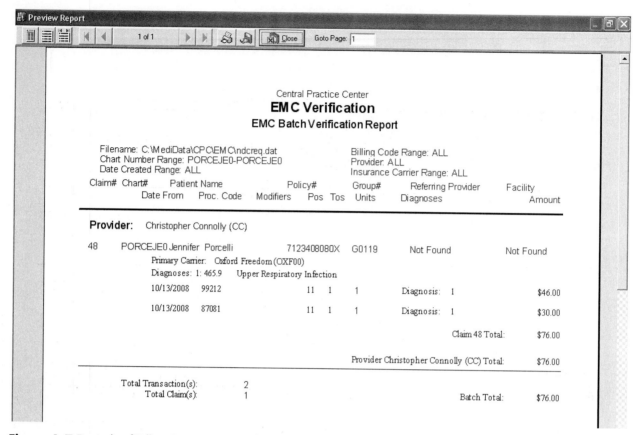

Figure 6–7 Example of Billing Program Screen for Claim Transmission   *Courtesy NDCMedisoft*

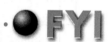

To ensure clean claims, software programs called claim scrubbers are used in many offices. They make sure that all required fields are filled and that only valid codes are used.

Direct Transmission

Some providers and payers exchange transactions directly. This method might be worth the expense of setting up for a practice's major payers, like Medicare.

Direct Data Entry (DDE)

Another option is DDE, in which the office uses an Internet-based service connected to the payer into which the claim's data elements are keyed. Like direct transmission, this method involves a high level of technical knowledge and investment at the medical office.

PREPARING PAPER CLAIMS

If a CMS-1500 (HCFA-1500) paper claim is required, it is prepared as summarized in Table 6-5 on pages 106–108. Figure 6-8 shows an example of this claim form. The CMS-1500 contains thirty-three form locators, which are numbered items. Form locators 1 through 13 refer to the patient and the patient's insurance coverage. Form locators 14 through 33 contain information about the provider and the transaction information, including the diagnoses, procedures, and charges. The claim is printed and sent to the payer.

APPROVED OMB-0938-0008

CARRIER

□□□ PICA

HEALTH INSURANCE CLAIM FORM

PICA □□□

1. MEDICARE	MEDICAID	CHAMPUS	CHAMPVA	GROUP HEALTH PLAN	FECA BLK LUNG	OTHER	1a. INSURED'S I.D. NUMBER	(FOR PROGRAM IN ITEM 1)
□ (Medicare #)	□ (Medicaid #)	□ (Sponsor's SSN)	□ (VA File #)	□ (SSN or ID)	□ (SSN)	□ (ID)		

3. PATIENT'S BIRTH DATE   MM   DD   YY   SEX   M □   F □

4. INSURED'S NAME (Last Name, First Name, Middle Initial)

5. PATIENT'S ADDRESS (No., Street)

6. PATIENT RELATIONSHIP TO INSURED   Self □   Spouse □   Child □   Other □

7. INSURED'S ADDRESS (No., Street)

CITY   STATE

8. PATIENT STATUS   Single □   Married □   Other □

CITY   STATE

ZIP CODE   TELEPHONE (Include Area Code)   (   )

Employed □   Full-Time Student □   Part-Time Student □

ZIP CODE   TELEPHONE (INCLUDE AREA CODE)   (   )

9. OTHER INSURED'S NAME (Last Name, First Name, Middle Initial)

10. IS PATIENT'S CONDITION RELATED TO:

11. INSURED'S POLICY GROUP OR FECA NUMBER

a. OTHER INSURED'S POLICY OR GROUP NUMBER

a. EMPLOYMENT? (CURRENT OR PREVIOUS)   □ YES   □ NO

a. INSURED'S DATE OF BIRTH   MM   DD   YY   SEX   M □   F □

b. OTHER INSURED'S DATE OF BIRTH   MM   DD   YY   SEX   M □   F □

b. AUTO ACCIDENT?   PLACE (State)   □ YES   □ NO

b. EMPLOYER'S NAME OR SCHOOL NAME

c. EMPLOYER'S NAME OR SCHOOL NAME

c. OTHER ACCIDENT?   □ YES   □ NO

c. INSURANCE PLAN NAME OR PROGRAM NAME

d. INSURANCE PLAN NAME OR PROGRAM NAME

10d. RESERVED FOR LOCAL USE

d. IS THERE ANOTHER HEALTH BENEFIT PLAN?   □ YES   □ NO   **If yes**, return to and complete item 9 a-d.

READ BACK OF FORM BEFORE COMPLETING & SIGNING THIS FORM.

12. PATIENT'S OR AUTHORIZED PERSON'S SIGNATURE I authorize the release of any medical or other information necessary to process this claim. I also request payment of government benefits either to myself or to the party who accepts assignment below.

SIGNED _____   DATE _____

13. INSURED'S OR AUTHORIZED PERSON'S SIGNATURE I authorize payment of medical benefits to the undersigned physician or supplier for services described below.

SIGNED _____

PATIENT AND INSURED INFORMATION

14. DATE OF CURRENT: MM   DD   YY   ◄ ILLNESS (First symptom) OR INJURY (Accident) OR PREGNANCY (LMP)

15. IF PATIENT HAS HAD SAME OR SIMILAR ILLNESS, GIVE FIRST DATE   MM   DD   YY

16. DATES PATIENT UNABLE TO WORK IN CURRENT OCCUPATION   FROM   MM   DD   YY   TO   MM   DD   YY

17. NAME OF REFERRING PHYSICIAN OR OTHER SOURCE

17a. I.D. NUMBER OF REFERRING PHYSICIAN

18. HOSPITALIZATION DATES RELATED TO CURRENT SERVICES   FROM   MM   DD   YY   TO   MM   DD   YY

19. RESERVED FOR LOCAL USE

20. OUTSIDE LAB?   □ YES   □ NO $ CHARGES

21. DIAGNOSIS OR NATURE OF ILLNESS OR INJURY. (RELATE ITEMS 1,2,3, OR 4 TO ITEM 24E BY LINE)

1. |___ . ___   3. |___ . ___

2. |___ . ___   4. |___ . ___

22. MEDICAID RESUBMISSION CODE   ORIGINAL REF. NO.

23. PRIOR AUTHORIZATION NUMBER

24. A DATE(S) OF SERVICE		B Place of Service	C Type of Service	D PROCEDURES, SERVICES, OR SUPPLIES (Explain Unusual Circumstances)	E DIAGNOSIS CODE	F $ CHARGES	G DAYS OR UNITS	H EPSDT Family Plan	I EMG	J COB	K RESERVED FOR LOCAL USE
From MM DD YY	To MM DD YY			CPT/HCPCS MODIFIER							
1											
2											
3											
4											
5											
6											

25. FEDERAL TAX I.D. NUMBER   SSN □ EIN □

26. PATIENT'S ACCOUNT NO.

27. ACCEPT ASSIGNMENT? (For govt. claims, see back)   □ YES   □ NO

28. TOTAL CHARGE $

29. AMOUNT PAID $

30. BALANCE DUE $

31. SIGNATURE OF PHYSICIAN OR SUPPLIER INCLUDING DEGREES OR CREDENTIALS (I certify that the statements on the reverse apply to this bill and are made a part thereof.)

SIGNED _____   DATE _____

32. NAME AND ADDRESS OF FACILITY WHERE SERVICES WERE RENDERED (if other than home or office)

33. PHYSICIAN'S OR SUPPLIER'S NAME, ADDRESS, ZIP CODE & TELEPHONE NO.

PIN#   GRP#

PHYSICIAN OR SUPPLIER INFORMATION

(APPROVED BY AMA COUNCIL ON MEDICAL SERVICE 8/88)

PLEASE PRINT OR TYPE

FORM HCFA-1500 (12-90)
FORM OWCP-1500   FORM RRB-1500

Figure 6-8 CMS-1500 Claim Form

Table 6-5 CMS-1500 Completion

Form Locator	Content
1	Type of Insurance: Medicare, Medicaid, TRICARE (labeled CHAMPUS), CHAMPVA, FECA Black Lung, Group Health Plan, or Other.
1a	Insured's ID Number: The insurance identification number that appears on the insurance card of the policyholder.
2	Patient's Name: As it appears on the insurance card.
3	Patient's Birth Date/Sex: Date of birth with year in four-digit format; appropriate selection for male or female.
4	Insured's Name: The full name of the person who holds the insurance policy (the insured). If the patient is a dependent, the insured may be a spouse, parent, or other person. If the insured is the patient, enter "Same."
5	Patient's Address: Address includes the number and street, city, state, and ZIP code.
6	Patient's Relationship to Insured: Self, spouse, child, or other.
7	Insured's Address: Address of the person who is listed in form locator 4. If the insured's address is the same as the patient's, enter "Same" in form locator 7. This form locator does not need to be completed if the patient is the insured person.
8	Patient Status: Marital status—single, married, or other—as well as the patient's employment status—employed, full-time student, or part-time student.
9	Other Insured's Name: If there is additional insurance coverage, the insured's name.
9a	Other Insured's Policy or Group Number: The policy or group number of the other insurance plan.
9b	Other Insured's Date of Birth: Date of birth and sex of the other insured.
9c	Employer's Name or School Name: Other insured's employer or school.
9d	Insurance Plan Name or Program Name: Other insured's insurance plan or program name.
10a–10c	Is Patient Condition Related to: To indicate whether the patient's condition is the result of a work injury, an automobile accident, or another type of accident. If the services provided are related to one of these occurrences, indicate this by marking yes. If the services are related to an automobile accident, enter the two-character abbreviation of the name of the state where the accident occurred. Other refers to injuries or conditions that can be reported to a liability insurance carrier or no-fault insurance program.
10d	Reserved for Local Use: Varies with the insurance plan.
11	Insured's Policy Group or FECA Number: As it appears on the insurance identification card.
11a	Insured's Date of Birth/Sex: The insured's date of birth and sex if the patient is not the insured.
11b	Employer's Name or School Name: Insured's employer or school.
11c	Insurance Plan Name or Program Name: Of the insured.

11d	Is There Another Health Benefit Plan? Yes if the patient is covered by additional insurance. If yes, form locators 9a–9d and/or 11–11c must also be completed. If the patient does not have additional insurance, select No. If not known, leave blank.
12	Patient's or Authorized Person's Signature: If the patient's or authorized representative's signature authorizing release of information is on file, the words "Signature on file" or "SOF" are entered in form locator 12. If an authorized representative is used because the patient is unable to sign, the representative's relationship to the patient and the reason the patient cannot sign are also entered in form locator 12.
13	Insured or Authorized Person's Signature: Indicating that the patient or patient's representative authorizes payments from the insurance carrier to be made directly to the provider of the services listed on the claim form.
14	Date of Current Illness or Injury or Pregnancy: The date that symptoms first began for the current illness, injury, or pregnancy. For pregnancy, enter the date of the patient's last menstrual period (LMP). If the actual date is not known, leave blank.
15	If Patient Has Had Same or Similar Illness: Date when the patient first consulted the provider for treatment of the same or a similar condition. If the patient has not had a same or similar illness, or if it is not known, leave blank.
16	Dates Patient Unable to Work in Current Occupation: Dates the patient has been unable to work in form locator 16. If not known, leave blank.
17	Name of Referring Physician or Other Source: Name of the physician or other source who referred the patient to the billing provider.
17a	ID Number of Referring Physician: Identifying number for the referring physician.
18	Hospitalization Dates Related to Current Services: If the services provided are needed because of a related hospitalization, the admission and discharge dates are entered. For patients still hospitalized, the admission date is listed in the From box, and the To box is left blank.
19	Reserved for Local Use.
20	Outside Lab? Varies with carrier.
21	Diagnosis or Nature of Illness or Injury: ICD-9-CM codes in priority order.
22	Medicaid Resubmission: Medicaid-specific.
23	Prior Authorization Number: If required by the carrier.
24A	Dates of Service: If the same service is provided multiple times, list the To and From dates once, and indicate the number of days or units in form locator 24G. If services were provided on a single day, the entry in form locator 24A varies with each carrier; some require the date in both the To and From columns; some require just the To column to be completed, and others require just the From column to be completed.
24B	Place of Service: A place of service (POS) code describes the location at which the service was provided.

24C	Type of Service: Carrier-specific code.
24D	Procedures, Services, or Supplies: CPT/HCPCS codes for services provided. Up to three modifiers can be listed next to each code. If there are more than three modifiers, enter -99 and list the additional modifiers in form locator 19.
24E	Diagnosis Code: Using the numbers (1, 2, 3, 4) listed to the left of the diagnosis codes in form locator 21, enter the diagnosis for each service listed in form locator 24D.
24F	$ Charges: For each service listed in form locator 24D, enter charges without dollar signs and decimals.
24G	Days or Units: The number of days or units.
24H	EPSDT Family Plan: Medicaid-specific.
24I	EMG (Emergency): If services were provided in an emergency room.
24J	COB (Coordination of Benefits): Some insurance plans require a check in this box if the patient has other insurance coverage in addition to the primary plan.
24K	Reserved for Local Use.
25	National Provider Identifier (NPI) when available, or tax or other ID.
26	Patient's Account No.: Patient account number used by the practice's accounting system.
27	Accept Assignment? If the physician accepts assignment, select Yes.
28	Total Charge: Total of all charges in form locator 24F.
29	Amount Paid: Amount of the patient payment that is applied to the services listed on this claim. If there is also payment from another insurance carrier, a copy of the remittance advice or claim denial should be forwarded. If no payment was made, enter none or 0.00.
30	Balance Due: Balance resulting from subtracting the amount in form locator 29 from the amount in form locator 28.
31	Signature of Physician or Supplier Including Degrees or Credentials: For claims that are sent using a computer, the provider's electronic signature appears. On claims that are printed and mailed, the provider's or supplier's signature, the date of the signature, and the provider's credentials (such as MD) are entered.
32	Name and Address of Facility Where Services Were Rendered (If Other Than Home or Office): If the facility and address where services were performed is the same as the one listed in form locator 33, enter "Same." If services were provided at a location other than the office or home, enter the name and address of the facility in form locator 32.
33	Physician's, Supplier's Billing Name, Address, ZIP code, and Telephone Number.

Chapter Summary

1. Medical billing programs are used in most medical offices to prepare health care claims. The program's databases are set up with data about the physicians, common diagnosis and procedure codes, fee schedules, and payers. To create a claim, the medical insurance specialist (a) records the patient's information, based on a new or updated patient information form, and determines the primary plan; (b) records services, charges, and payments based on the patient's encounter form; and (c) instructs the program to create and transmit the claim.

2. The five major sections and contents of the HIPAA claim are: (a) provider information, including the billing and the pay-to provider addresses and NPIs; (b) the subscriber/patient information, including the subscriber (and the patient, if not the subscriber, with a relationship code) name and health plan number as they appear on the insurance card, address, identifiers, group or policy number, group or plan name, and a claim filing indictor code; (c) payer information for the destination payer, including name, ID, and an assignment of benefits code; (d) claim details, including the claim control number, total charges and patient payment, place of service code, diagnosis codes, and data elements about rendering or referring providers; and (e) service line information, including service line control numbers, date of service, procedure codes, charges, and diagnosis code links.

3. The unique claim control numbers and line item control numbers that are assigned by the sender are important because these numbers appear on payments and other transactions that are returned by payers.

4. Electronic claims can be transmitted by using a clearinghouse, by direct transmission, and by direct data entry (DDE). Most medical offices use clearinghouses to send their claims in HIPAA EDI format.

Check Your Understanding

Part 1. **In the space provided, write the word or phrase that best completes each sentence.**

_____ **1.** The HIPAA claim is a(n) _electronic_ claim, rather than a paper claim.

_____ **2.** EDI is an abbreviation for _electronic data interchange_

_____ **3.** Standard code sets are established by HIPAA's _EHTC_ _TCS_ provisions.

_____ **4.** A(n) _claim attachment_ is a document that accompanies a claim.

_____ **5.** After an insurance claim is completed, all entries must be _edited_.

_____ **6.** The three steps in the claim preparation process are recording patients' information; recording services, charges, and payments for patients' encounters; and _preparing_ and _transmitting_ claims to payers.

_____ **7.** The HIPAA _Security_ Rule sets standards for protecting PHI when it is maintained or transmitted electronically.

_____ **8.** The National Provider Identifier (NPI) has _10_ digits.

_____ **9.** Where patients received services is reported on the HIPAA claim with a _place of service_ code.

_____ **10.** An _Audit edit Claim response_ report is sent from a clearinghouse to the sender of a claim to ask for missing or incorrect information.

Part 2. **Determine the primary plan:**

A. George Rangley enrolled in the ACR plan in 2008 and in the New York Health plan in 2006.

George's primary plan: _New York plan_

B. Mary is the child of Gloria and Craig Bivilaque, who are divorced. Mary is a dependent under both Craig's and Gloria's plans. Gloria has custody of Mary.

Mary's primary plan: _Gloria_

C. Karen Kaplan's date of birth is 10/11/1970; her husband Carl was born on 12/8/1971. Their child Ralph was born on 4/15/2000. Ralph is a dependent under both Karen's and Carl's plans.

Ralph's primary plan: _Karens_

D. Belle Estaphan has medical insurance from Internet Services, from which she retired last year. She is on Medicare, but is also covered under her husband Bernard's plan from Orion International, where he works.

Belle's primary plan: _Medicare_

E. Jim Larenges is covered under his spouse's plan and also has medical insurance through his employer.

Jim's primary plan: _employer_

Part 3. Choose the letter of the best answer.

____ **1.** If a physician uses a billing service to prepare and transmit its health care claims, which entity is the pay-to provider?
    a. billing service
    b. physician
    c. referring provider

____ **2.** Medical billing programs store information such as patients' names in:
    a. transactions
    b. audit/edit reports
    c. databases

____ **3.** Medical offices restrict access to patients' protected health information by limiting it to those who:
    a. are staff members
    b. need the information
    c. process HIPAA claims

____ **4.** The name of the paper claim form is:
    a. HIPAA 837
    b. CMS-1492
    c. CMS-1500

____ **5.** Which format is required by CMS for Medicare claims?
    a. CMS-1500
    b. HIPAA claim
    c. neither a nor b

____ **6.** On a HIPAA claim, the line item control number is in the:
    a. claim information section
    b. provider information section
    c. services section

____ **7.** If the subscriber and the patient are not the same person, what type of code describes this?
    a. relationship code
    b. place of service code
    c. National Payer ID

____ **8.** Which type of code describes the medical specialty of a provider?
    a. pay-to code
    b. taxonomy code
    c. relationship code

____ **9.** How many diagnosis codes must appear for each service line?
    a. one
    b. two
    c. four

____ **10.** The predominant method for transmitting claims is:
    a. direct data entry (DDE)
    b. direct transmission
    c. via clearinghouse

Part 4. Supply the answers to the following cases.

A. Joan McNavish, a sixty-one-year-old retiree, is covered by her husband's insurance policy. Her husband, Ray, is still working and receives health benefits through his employer, Rockford Valley Concrete, which has a PPO plan. In this case, who is the subscriber and who is the patient?

Ray Subscriber; Joan is the patient

B. Sherry Denise Cleaver is a patient in the medical office where you work. This information appears on her patient information and encounter forms:

Name: Sherry Denise Cleaver
Established Patient
Birth Date: July 1, 2000
Marital Status: Single
Responsible Person: James T. Cleaver
Relationship to Patient: Father
Insured's Plan: BMA PPO

Diagnosis of otitis media, left, on May 13, 2008; the charge is $22 for a CPT 99211. The medical office collected a copayment of $10 and waits for payment directly from the insurance companies on assigned claims.

Supply the following data elements:
Subscriber: *James T. Cleaver*
Patient: *Sherry Denise Cleaver*
Relationship of Patient to Subscriber: *Father*
Claim Filing Indicator Code: *12?*
Total Charge: *$12*
Amount Collected: *$10*
Place of Service Code: *11*
Diagnosis Code: *382.9*
Date of Service: *5, 13, 08*
Procedure Code/Charge: *99211*

C. The following information appears on a series of encounter forms for patient Daniel M. Williams. You are preparing a claim for the three encounters.

Patient: Daniel M. Williams (EP)
Insurance: Aetna POS
Insured: Marla Y. Jones (grandmother)

Date: 6-14-08
T-101 P-90 R-18 BP 132/76 WT 175
CC: Swollen neck glands, fever, headache, general malaise since this morning
Dx: Epidemic parotitis.
Rx: Rest, fluids, Tylenol for headache prn. Return in 5 days for recheck.
Services and Charges: Office visit, problem-focused history and exam, straightforward decision making: $65

Date: 6-19-08
T-101 P-88 R-18 BP 130/60
CC: Fever, pain and swelling of right testicle.
Dx: Orchitis, complication of epidemic parotitis.
Rx: Ampicillin 500 mg. #16; IM Ampicillin 500 mg. Return 2 days for recheck.
Services and Charges: Office visit, problem-focused history and exam, straightforward decision making: $65
Intramuscular (IM) administration of antibiotic (Ampicillin) 500 mg, $20

Date: 6-21-08
T-98.8 P-80 R-16 BP 132/74
Rx: Recheck, improvement, continue meds, recheck in 2 weeks.
Dx: Orchitis.
Services and Charges: Office visit, problem-focused history and exam, straightforward decision making: $65

Supply the following data elements:
Subscriber: _Marla y jonas_
Patient: _Daniel M Williams_
Relationship: _grand mother_
Claim Filing Indicator Code: _13_
Total Charge: _$175_
Place of Service Code: _11_
Diagnosis Codes: _____

Service Line Information:
Date of Service: _6-14-08_
Procedure Code/Charge: _____
Diagnosis: _Epidemic parotitis_

Date of Service: _6-19-08_
Procedure Code/Charge: _____
Diagnosis: _Orchitis complication of epidemic parotitis_

Date of Service: _6-21-08_
Procedure Code/Charge: _____
Diagnosis: _Orchitis_

Date of Service: _____
Procedure Code/Charge: _____
Diagnosis: _____

```
  1
 65
 65
 65
 195
- 20
 175
```

D. The following information is in the file of patient Martha M. Butler. You are preparing a claim for the encounters.

Name: Martha M. Butler (EP)
Insurance Medicare Part B

Date: 4-19-2008
T-98.8 P-68 R-15 BP 178/98 WT 155
CC: This a.m. while going to get mail pt. fell on sidewalk; a neighbor brought her in c/o pain and disability in left hip area, SOB, chest pain.
Exam: Pt. in distress, X-ray L hip two views—negative, ECG T-wave inversion.
Lab: Cardiac enzymes, electrolytes.
Dx: Sprained L hip, essential hypertension, R/O angina pectoris.
Rx: Injection 2.0 cc Norflex IM, moist heat, Norflex tablets #12, Inderal capsules 80 mg #30.
Return in 3 days for lab results and recheck.

Date: 4-22-2008
T-98.6 P-68 R-15 BP 150/88
Lab Results: Within normal limits.
Exam: Hip improving, ECG negative.
Dx: Essential hypertension, angina pectoris.
Rx: Continue prescribed meds. Nitrostat tablets, one tab dissolved under tongue at first sign of angina attack.

List of Fees for Service:
Date: 4-19-2008
Dx: Sprained L hip, essential hypertension.
Services and Charges:
Office visit, detailed history and detailed exam, decision making of moderate complexity: $80
X-ray L hip, complete, two views, $90
Therapeutic Intramuscular Injection 2.0 cc Norflex IM, $12
ECG routine, 12 leads, interpretation and report, $55

Date: 4-22-2008
Dx: Essential hypertension, angina pectoris.
Services and Charges: Office visit, problem-focused history and exam, straightforward decision making: $65

Supply the following data elements:
Subscriber/Patient: _Martha M. Butler_
Claim Filing Indicator Code: _MB_
Total Charge: _$113_
Place of Service Code: _____
Diagnosis Codes: _____

Service Line Information
Date of Service: ____4-19-2008____

Procedure Code/Charge: _____

Diagnosis: _Sprained L hip, essential hypertension, R/O angina pectoris_

Date of Service: __4-22-2008____

Procedure Code/Charge: _____

Diagnosis: _Essential Hypertension angina pectoris_

Date of Service: __4-19-2008____

Procedure Code/Charge: _____

Diagnosis: _Sprained L hip, essential Hypertension_

Date of Service: ____4-22-08____

Procedure Code/Charge: _____

Diagnosis: _Essential Hypertension, angina pectoris_

Date of Service: _____

Procedure Code/Charge: _____

Diagnosis: _____

CHAPTER 7

Payment Follow-up and Collections

Objectives

After completing this chapter, you will be able to define the key terms and:

1. Describe the claim determination process used by health plans.
2. Follow five steps to process reimbursement advices (RAs) from health plans.
3. Discuss common reasons for and appeals of reduced or denied payments.
4. Describe the patient billing and collections process.
5. Handle patients' inquiries about insurance and billing problems.

Key Terms

accounts receivable	downcoding	patient ledger
adjustments	electronic funds transfer (EFT)	patient statement
appeal	insurance aging report	preexisting condition
determination	patient aging report	uncollectible account

Why This Chapter Is Important to You

The information in this chapter will enable you to:

- Solve common payment problems.
- Understand how health plans can help with questions about claims.
- Increase your confidence by learning to answer patients' common questions about claims and bills.
- Check payers' RAs for accurate and complete payment.
- Understand and explain explanation of benefits statements to patients.

What Do You Think?

One of the critical goals of a medical insurance specialist is to have claims approved and paid promptly by insurance carriers. Another goal is to help ensure prompt payments from patients. What steps can the specialist take to avoid claim rejection and to speed correct reimbursement from carriers and patients?

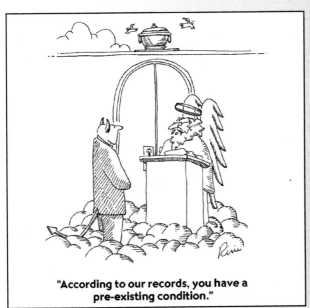

"According to our records, you have a pre-existing condition."

A major responsibility of the medical insurance specialist is the preparation and transmission of clean claims that will be paid in full and on time. Claims that payers pay late, decide not to pay, or pay at a reduced level have a negative effect on accounts receivable, the practice's cash flow. To follow up on claims, medical insurance specialists need to understand the process that payers follow to examine claims and determine payments. The flow of information in this process is shown in Figure 7-1.

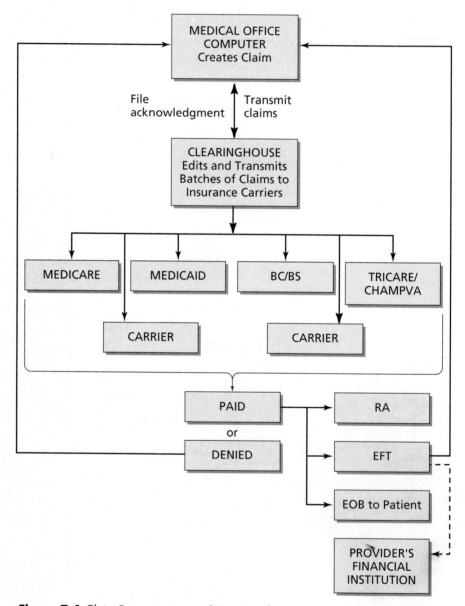

Figure 7–1 Claim Determination and Payment Flow

Claim Processing

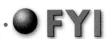
When a payer has accepted a health care claim as complete and on time, in keeping with the payer's rules for the time of submission, the claims department answers two major questions:

1. Whether benefits are due according to the patient's policy.
2. Whether the services provided were medically necessary.

The first items checked are the subscriber's and patient's policy identification numbers. Then the payer ensures that policy payments, such as premiums, are up-to-date and that the policy is in effect for the date of service. Correct spelling of names and use of names as they appear in the payer's master file are essential. A nickname or typographical error can make it very difficult to identify a person covered by a policy or contract.

The claim is reviewed by claims examiners and, sometimes, by a medical professional. Procedure codes are compared with the policy's schedule of benefits to see whether the reported services are covered. The examiner may decide to hold the claim and ask the treating physician for additional clinical information. In this case, the examiner may request documentation to check:

- Where the service took place
- Whether the treatments were appropriate and a logical outcome of the facts and conditions shown in the medical record
- That services provided were accurately reported

After the case is examined, a payment determination is made—a decision whether to (1) pay the claim, (2) deny the claim, or (3) reduce the payment for the claim. If the claims examiner decides that the claim falls within normal guidelines and is complete, the claim is paid. If it is complete but not reimbursable, the claim is denied. If the examiner determines that any of the services the patient received were at too high a level for the related diagnosis, the examiner may assign a lower-level code to the service and pay a lower amount than was billed.

Reduced Payments for Claims

When the level of service is reduced by the claims examiner—called downcoding—it is because the procedure does not link correctly to the diagnosis. Perhaps the procedure's place of service is an emergency department, but the patient's problem is not considered an emergency. Claims may also be downcoded because the documentation fails to support the level of service claimed. For example, if the physician has coded a high-level evaluation and management service for a patient who presents with an apparently straightforward problem, the claims examiner is likely to request the encounter documentation. The medical record should contain information about the type of medical history and examination done as well as the complexity of the medical decision making that was performed. If the documentation does not support the service, the examiner downcodes the E/M code to a level considered appropriate.

Denied Claims

Claims may be denied because the services are not covered by the patient's contract with the insurance carrier. Common examples are when the patient's diagnosis is a preexisting condition—one that existed before the insured's contract went into effect. Some policies require a waiting period before preexisting conditions are covered. An excluded illness or disorder is one that is specified in the policy as not covered. The insurance carrier will not pay for services for preexisting conditions or exclusions, but the physician may bill the patient for them.

When payment is denied, both the physician and the patient are notified by the insurance carrier. The medical insurance specialist should follow up with a letter to the patient explaining what action is being taken. In cases of preexisting conditions and canceled coverage, the patient is responsible for the bill. Any specific written correspondence received from the insurance company should be filed with the patient's records. If the patient has questions, the information from the insurance company may help resolve them.

Overdue Claims

Just as medical offices are required to file claims within a certain period of time, health plans have contractual agreements to pay claims within a period of time from receipt. Claims must be monitored until payments are received. Most offices follow up on claim status seven to fourteen days after claims are transmitted.

To avoid late payments, medical insurance specialists regularly review the insurance aging report. This report shows the ages of unpaid claims—that is, how long after the dates of claims payers have taken to respond to them (see Figure 7-2).

In addition to regular claim follow-up, other reasons for contacting the insurance carrier are:

- The carrier notifies the medical office that a claim is being investigated. This might be due to preexisting conditions, workers' compensation, or other reasons. After a period of thirty days from this notice, however, follow-up should be done.

- An unclear denial of payment or an incorrect payment is received.

- Payment is received with no indication of the amount of the allowed charge or how much the patient is responsible for.

- The carrier asks for more information to process the claim. For example, a claim may contain an unlisted CPT code. In response, the payer asks for a special report (a narrative description) on the procedure or precise details of the service provided.

HIPAA Tip

Medical offices use a HIPAA transaction called the claim status inquiry to electronically follow up with payers. The payer responds with the status of the claim.

Primary Insurance Aging
As of 11/30/2008

Date of Service	Procedure	-- Past -- 0 - 30	-- Past -- 31 - 60	-- Past -- 61 - 90	-- Past -- 91 - 120	-- Past -- 121 ---->	Total Balance

Aetna Choice (AET00)   (555)777-1000

WILLIWA0   Walter Williams   **SS: 401-26-9939**   **Policy: ABC103562239**   **Group: BDC1001**
Birthdate: 9/4/1936

Claim: 53   Initial Billing Date: 10/8/2008   Last Billing Date: 10/8/2008

Date of Service	Procedure	0 - 30	31 - 60	61 - 90	91 - 120	121 ---->	Total Balance
10/1/2008	99212		46.00				46.00
10/1/2008	93000		70.00				70.00
		0.00	116.00	0.00	0.00	0.00	116.00
	Insurance Totals	$0.00	$116.00	$0.00	$0.00	$0.00	$116.00

Anthem BCBS PPO (ANT01)   (555)888-1000

CARUTRO0   Robin Caruthers   **SS: 331-24-0789**   **Policy: GH331240789**   **Group: OH4071**
Birthdate: 3/29/1979

Claim: 49   Initial Billing Date: 10/6/2008   Last Billing Date: 10/6/2008

Date of Service	Procedure	0 - 30	31 - 60	61 - 90	91 - 120	121 ---->	Total Balance
10/6/2008	99212		46.00				46.00
		0.00	46.00	0.00	0.00	0.00	46.00
	Insurance Totals	$0.00	$46.00	$0.00	$0.00	$0.00	$46.00

Cigna HMO Plus (CIG00)   (555)666-3001

PEREZCA0   Carmen Perez   **SS: 140-24-6113**   **Policy: 140603312X**
Birthdate: 5/15/1934

Claim: 52   Initial Billing Date: 10/8/2008   Last Billing Date: 10/8/2008

Date of Service	Procedure	0 - 30	31 - 60	61 - 90	91 - 120	121 ---->	Total Balance
10/1/2008	99213		62.00				62.00
		0.00	62.00	0.00	0.00	0.00	62.00
	Insurance Totals	$0.00	$62.00	$0.00	$0.00	$0.00	$62.00

Figure 7-2 Example of Insurance Aging Report

Professional Focus

PROCESSING THE REMITTANCE ADVICE

The remittance advice (RA) sent by the payer to the medical office summarizes the determinations for a number of claims. See Figure 7-3 for an example of an RA received by a medical office. (The explanation of benefits the patient receives covers just the patient's determination, as shown in Figure 1-4 on page 12.) The RA lists the claim control number, patient, dates of service, types of service, and charges. It also describes the way the amount of the benefit payment was determined. RAs usually cover claims for a number of patients, and the payments may not be for every service line on a particular claim.

When a RA is received, usually electronically, the medical insurance specialist reviews it for accuracy and completeness. The medical billing program is used to locate each claim listed on the RA, following these steps:

1. Match the claim control number, patient's name, and date of service with the payer's payments.

2. Check the patient data, plan, and listed procedures against the claim. Note any mismatched or missing information so that the claim can be corrected.

3. Compare the payment for each procedure with the expected amount. If a physician participates in the plan, the difference between what the physician charged on the claim and the allowed charge may be described as disallowed, nonallowed, not eligible for payment, or a similar phrase. This disallowed amount may be listed as a separate item. If not, it can be calculated by subtracting the allowed charge from the amount the physician charged.

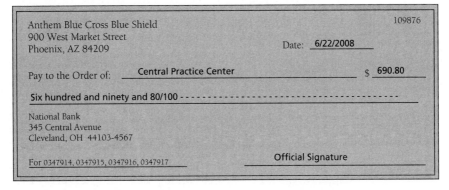

PROVIDER REMITTANCE

Anthem Blue Cross Blue Shield
900 West Market Street
Phoenix, AZ 84209

Date: 6/22/2008

	Patient's name	Dates of service from - thru	POS	Proc	Qty	Charge amount	Allowed amount	Patient coins.	Amt paid provider	Patient balance
	Claim number 0347914									
4-101	Daiute, Angelo X	06/17/08 - 06/17/08	11	36415	1	$11.00	$8.00	$1.60	$6.40	$1.60
4-102	Daiute, Angelo X	06/17/08 - 06/17/08	11	80050	1	$98.00	$90.00	$9.00	$81.00	$9.00
4-103	Daiute, Angelo X	06/17/08 - 06/17/08	11	81000	1	$12.00	$10.00	$1.00	$9.00	$1.00
4-104	Daiute, Angelo X	06/17/08 - 06/17/08	11	93000	1	$51.00	$50.00	$5.00	$45.00	$5.00
4-105	Daiute, Angelo X	06/17/08 - 06/17/08	11	99386	1	$123.00	$76.00	$15.20	$60.80	$15.20
										31.80
	Claim number 0347915									
5-101	Daiute, Brian G	06/17/08 - 06/17/08	11	99383	1	$98.00	$90.00	$9.00	$81.00	$9.00
5-102	Daiute, Brian G	06/17/08 - 06/17/08	11	90711	1	$74.00	$70.00	$14.00	$56.00	$14.00
										$23.00
	Claim number 0347916									
6-101	Daiute, Mary F	06/17/08 - 06/17/08	11	36415	1	$11.00	$8.00	$1.60	$6.40	$1.60
6-102	Daiute, Mary F	06/17/08 - 06/17/08	11	80050	1	$98.00	$90.00	$9.00	$81.00	$9.00
6-103	Daiute, Mary F	06/17/08 - 06/17/08	11	81000	1	$12.00	$10.00	0.00	$10.00	0.00
6-104	Daiute, Mary F	06/17/08 - 06/17/08	11	93000	1	$51.00	$50.00	$5.00	$45.00	$5.00
6-105	Daiute, Mary F	06/17/08 - 06/17/08	11	99386	1	$123.00	$76.00	$15.20	$60.80	$15.20
6-106	Daiute, Mary F	06/17/08 - 06/17/08	11	88150	1	$212.00	$212.00	0.00	0.00	$212.00**
										$242.80
	Claim number 0347917									
7-101	Daiute, Rosemary B	06/17/08 - 06/17/08	11	99384	1	$122.00	$64.00	$12.80	$51.20	$12.80
7-102	Daiute, Rosemary B	06/17/08 - 06/17/08	11	90707	1	$82.00	$82.00	$8.20	$73.80	$8.20
7-103	Daiute, Rosemary B	06/17/08 - 06/17/08	11	90702	1	$30.00	$26.00	$2.60	$23.40	$2.60
										$23.60

**Total for patient exceeds annual maximum for DME.

* * * * * * * * Check #109876 is attached in the amount of $690.80 * * * * * * * *

Anthem Blue Cross Blue Shield
900 West Market Street
Phoenix, AZ 84209

109876

Date: 6/22/2008

Pay to the Order of: Central Practice Center $ 690.80

Six hundred and ninety and 80/100 -

National Bank
345 Central Avenue
Cleveland, OH 44103-4567

For 0347914, 0347915, 0347916, 0347917   Official Signature

Figure 7–3 Example of Remittance Advice and Payment

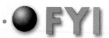
4. Read the carrier's explanations for unpaid, reduced, or denied claims. If the carrier's action is not warranted, the claim may be resubmitted or appealed, as described later in this chapter.

5. Determine the amounts of any write-offs that must be entered as adjustments in the patient's account. Also note the balance due from the patient or refund due to the patient (if the patient paid in advance or overpaid on the account).

Payment deposit is handled according to office practices. It may be a check or a notice of an electronic deposit called an electronic funds transfer (EFT). This type of payment is deposited directly in the practice's bank account.

If the patient has not assigned benefits to the provider, a benefits statement and the payment are sent directly to the patient. Even if no payment is due, a benefits explanation is usually sent. For example, if the physician's charges were applied to the patient's deductible, the physician does not receive a check. However, the health plan still sends a benefits statement.

APPEALS

When an incorrect payment is received, the carrier should be contacted. The carrier may have made a mistake and not entered the code that was submitted, which requires an adjustment to the payment. Sometimes, instead of a routine error, the carrier's reimbursement for services is considered inadequate or incorrect by the physician. In either case, a claim rejection can be appealed. A claim appeal is a written request for a review of payment. It is a formal way of asking the insurance carrier to reconsider its claim determination.

An appeal is usually filed in the following situations:

- The physician did not file for preauthorization in a timely manner due to unusual circumstances.

- The physician thinks that the payment received for a procedure is inadequate.

- The physician disagrees with the carrier's decision about a patient's preexisting condition.

- A patient has unusual circumstances that affect medical treatment.

A letter requesting an appeal of an inadequate payment might be worded as follows: "I am requesting special reconsideration of the disallowance for patient Mary Amamot, Case #1728564. A copy of the RA is enclosed for your review. I am also enclosing a list of fees that our research determined other plans allow for this CPT code. Your maximum allowed fees are below what comparable plans pay. We are certain our fees are cost-efficient and are based on the current relative value. Please inform us of your decision by calling or writing. We will contact you if we have not received an answer within thirty days."

If, after an appeal, the health plan denies what the physician considers fair compensation for services, the physician may want a peer review, in which an objective, unbiased group of physicians determines what payment is adequate for services provided. Another level of appeal is directed to the state's insurance commissioner. Each state has such a regulatory agency for the insurance industry, which is a liaison between the patient and the health plan, and between the physician and the health plan. Physician, health plan, or patient may appeal to the insurance commissioner if any of the three feels unfairly treated.

PATIENT BILLING AND COLLECTIONS

When the patient completes an office visit, the medical insurance specialist enters the transactions in the medical billing program. As patients' charges and payments are posted, the billing program also updates the patient ledger, or patient account record, a collection of all the financial activity in each patient's account. Later, when insurance payments are received for patients, those payments are also posted to the patient's account and reduce the balance that the patient owes. If a secondary insurance plan is involved, the payment information is transmitted to that payer, and any resulting payments on the patient's behalf are also posted.

If the physician has not accepted assignment and is not going to file a claim for a patient, patients are usually required to pay at the end of the visit. When the physician accepts assignment and is going to file a claim, the patient does not usually pay fees, other than any required copayment or deductible, at the time of service. The amount of the copayment is entered and subtracted from the balance due. Then the health care claim for the service is created and transmitted to the payer.

Patients' Statements

Patients owe amounts corresponding to their health plan coverage. A patient may owe a coinsurance payment. Patients also owe for services not covered by the policy. For these, the amount due from the patient is the amount that the physician charged—the usual fee. Since the services are not under contract, no allowed charges are in effect. The patient owes the entire physician's fee, which the physician may collect from the patient.

After all payer payments have been received on a claim, the medical insurance specialist uses the medical billing program to update patient statements, or bills. These patient statements are mailed to patients who have balances due on their accounts after insurance payments have been received. Practices usually prepare patient statements to be mailed on a regular basis. For example, twice a week bills are sent to a certain group of patients, such as selected alphabetically. This way of billing, called cycle billing, might be set up as follows: Monday, last names beginning with A through D, Wednesday E through H, the following Monday, I though L, and so on.

Follow the example of patient Karen Giroux, with a visit on October 7, 2008, and an RA posted on October 8, 2008. Figure 7-4 (on page 126) shows the transaction screen of the medical billing program after the visit has been posted. Figure 7-5 (on page 126) shows the ledger, illustrating the entry of the transactions for the office visit and the payment. The patient statement shown in Figure 7-6 (on page 127) is sent to the patient and shows the balance that is owed. When patient payments are received, they are recorded in the billing program.

> ✔ **Compliance Tip**
>
> Transactions should not be deleted in the patient billing program, because doing so could be interpreted by an auditor as a fraudulent act. Instead, corrections, changes, and write-offs are made with **adjustments** to existing transactions. The adjusting entries give both the medical office and the patient a history of events in case there is a billing inquiry or an audit.

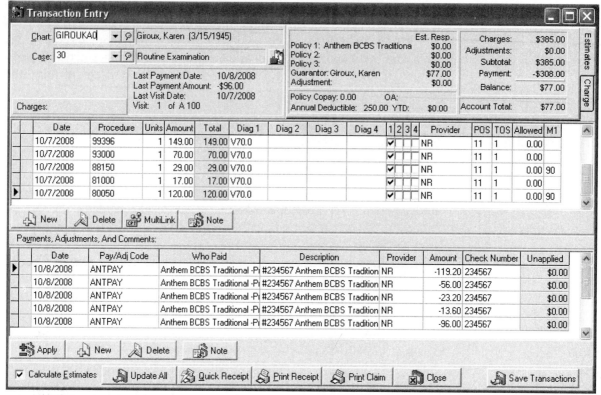

Figure 7–4 Transaction Screen

Posting Payment

Valley Associates, P.C.
Patient Account Ledger
As of October 31, 2008

Entry	Date	POS	Description	Procedure	Document	Provider	Amount
GIROUKA0	**Karen Giroux**			(555)683-5364			
	Last Payment:	-96.00	On: 10/8/2008				
6	10/7/2008			99396	0310060000	NR	149.00
7	10/7/2008			93000	0310060000	NR	70.00
8	10/7/2008			88150	0310060000	NR	29.00
9	10/7/2008			81000	0310060000	NR	17.00
10	10/7/2008			80050	0310060000	NR	120.00
40	10/8/2008		#234567 Anthem BCBS Traditiona	ANTPAY	0310060000	NR	-119.20
41	10/8/2008		#234567 Anthem BCBS Traditiona	ANTPAY	0310060000	NR	-56.00
42	10/8/2008		#234567 Anthem BCBS Traditiona	ANTPAY	0310060000	NR	-23.20
43	10/8/2008		#234567 Anthem BCBS Traditiona	ANTPAY	0310060000	NR	-13.60
44	10/8/2008		#234567 Anthem BCBS Traditiona	ANTPAY	0310060000	NR	-96.00
	Patient Totals						77.00
	Ledger Totals						77.00

Figure 7–5 Patient Ledger

Showing Payments

Valley Associates, P.C.
1400 West Center Street
Toledo, OH 43601-0123
(555)321-0987

Statement Date
10/31/2008

Page
1

Karen Giroux
14A West Front St
Brooklyn, OH 44144-1234

Chart Number
GIROUKA0

Date	Document	Description	Case Number	Amount
			Previous Balance:	0.00

Patient: Karen Giroux   Chart #: GIROUKA0
  Case Description: Routine Examination Date of Last Payment: 10/8/2008   Amount: -96.00

Date	Document	Description	Case Number	Amount
10/7/2008	0310060000	EP Prev 40-64	30	149.00
10/7/2008	0310060000	ECG Complete	30	70.00
10/7/2008	0310060000	Pap Smear	30	29.00
10/7/2008	0310060000	Urinalysis	30	17.00
10/7/2008	0310060000	General Health Panel	30	120.00
10/8/2008	0310060000	Anthem BCBS Traditional Payment	30	-119.20
10/8/2008	0310060000	Anthem BCBS Traditional Payment	30	-56.00
10/8/2008	0310060000	Anthem BCBS Traditional Payment	30	-23.20
10/8/2008	0310060000	Anthem BCBS Traditional Payment	30	-13.60
10/8/2008	0310060000	Anthem BCBS Traditional Payment	30	-96.00

Total Charges	Total Payments	Total Adjustments	Balance Due
$385.00	-$308.00	$0.00	77.00

Figure 7–6 Patient Statement

The Collection Process

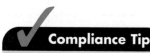
The collection process really begins with effective communications with patients about their responsibility to pay for services. When patients understand the charges and agree to pay them in advance, collecting the payments is not usually a problem. Most patients pay their bills on time. However, every practice has some patients who do not pay their bills when they receive their monthly statements. Patients' reasons for not paying range from forgetfulness or inability to pay to dissatisfaction with the services or charges.

Medical insurance specialists are often responsible for collections from patients. The patient aging report printed by the patient billing program is the starting point, since it shows which patients' payments are due or overdue (termed *past due*). Figure 7-7 shows an example of a patient aging report. The aging begins on the date of the bill. For each account, an aging report shows the name of the patient, the last payment, and the amount of charges in each of these categories:

- *Current:* 0 to 30 days
- *Past:* 31 to 60 days
- *Past:* 61 to 90 days
- *Past:* Over 91 days

Each office sets its own procedures for the collection process. Large bills have priority over smaller ones. Usually, an automatic reminder notice and a second statement are mailed when a bill has not been paid thirty days after it was issued. Some medical offices phone a patient with a thirty-day overdue account. If the bill is not then paid, a series of collection letters is generated at intervals, each more stringent in its tone and more direct in its approach. Some medical offices use small claims court or outside collection agencies to pursue significant unpaid bills.

Writing Off Uncollectible Accounts

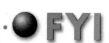

- If patients have large bills that they must pay over time, a financial arrangement for a series of payments may be made. Such arrangements may be governed by specific laws in each state.
- If the practice's printed or displayed payment policy covers adding finance charges on late accounts, it is acceptable to do so. The amount of the finance charge must comply with federal and state law.

If no payment has been made after the collection process, the medical insurance specialist follows the office policy on bills it does not expect to collect. Usually, if all collection attempts have been exhausted and it would cost more to continue pursuing payment than the amount to be collected, the process is ended. In this case, the amount is called an uncollectible account or bad debt and is written off from the expected revenues.

Patient Aging

As of November 30, 2008

Chart	Name	Birthdate	Current 0 - 30	Past 31 - 60	Past 61 - 90	Past 91 ----->	Total Balance
CARUTRO0 Last Pmt: -20.00	Robin Caruthers On: 10/6/2008	3/29/1979 (555)629-0222		46.00			46.00
ESTEPWI0 Last Pmt: -22.40	Wilma Estephan On: 10/8/2008	3/14/1940 (555)683-5272		5.60			5.60
GIROUKA0 Last Pmt: -96.00	Karen Giroux On: 10/8/2008	3/15/1945 (555)683-5364		77.00			77.00
PEREZCA0 Last Pmt: -20.00	Carmen Perez On: 10/1/2008	5/15/1934 (555)692-3314			62.00		62.00
PORCEJE0 Last Pmt: -15.00	Jennifer Porcelli On: 10/13/2008	7/5/1970 (555)709-0388		76.00			76.00
WILLIWA0 Last Pmt: -15.00	Walter Williams On: 10/1/2008	9/4/1936 (555)936-0216			116.00		116.00
	Report Aging Totals		$0.00	$204.60	$178.00	$0.00	382.60
	Percent of Aging Total		0.0 %	53.5 %	46.5 %	0.0 %	100.00 %

Figure 7-7 Example of Patient Aging Report

Communicating with Patients

Patients with complaints and problems with their health plans often need a go-between to contact the carrier and get questions answered. A medical insurance specialist with expertise and objectivity can build good will for the physician's office by using problem solving and communication skills to fulfill this role. The first step in answering patients' inquiries about claims is to find out exactly what the problem is. Ask the patient whether he or she has:

- Contacted the health plan
- Talked to the service representative
- Reviewed the policy

Often, the answer is no. The patient may not understand the insurance policy or may be confused about the rules of an HMO. On other occasions, the payer has made an error, and the patient is correct.

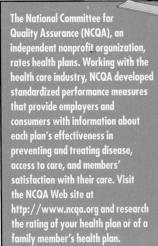

Explore the Internet

The National Committee for Quality Assurance (NCQA), an independent nonprofit organization, rates health plans. Working with the health care industry, NCQA developed standardized performance measures that provide employers and consumers with information about each plan's effectiveness in preventing and treating disease, access to care, and members' satisfaction with their care. Visit the NCQA Web site at http://www.ncqa.org and research the rating of your health plan or of a family member's health plan.

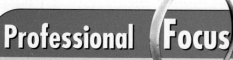

Professional Focus

Career Opportunities in Collections

Collection specialists in medical offices are employed to ensure receipt of the greatest possible percentage of fees owed by payers and patients. In a small medical office, a collection specialist may be a part of the billing staff. In a large group practice, a separate collection department may be set up to focus just on this important function.

Patients understandably get upset when they receive unexpected large bills or an incorrect payment, or when there is a delayed payment. The medical insurance specialist is the patients' advocate with the health plan. Sometimes the problem is just a misunderstanding because the patient does not know the right questions to ask, does not understand the answers, or is unaware that benefits have changed. In other situations, the patient may accuse the office staff of billing incorrectly. In these cases, try to listen carefully for the facts without letting feelings interfere.

If the patient has already called the health plan but is still upset or confused, the medical insurance specialist should call again and listen carefully to the explanation. The patient may have been too stressed to understand it. Explaining the solution again to the patient may help clear up misunderstandings.

Following are some techniques to use when explaining insurance issues to patients:

- Volunteer to explain. Speak slowly and calmly.
- Use simple language. Try to avoid insurance jargon.
- Explain more than once when necessary.
- Ask the patient, "Do you understand?" or say, "Perhaps I can explain that better."
- Remember, patients are under stress. Use respect and care.

Chapter Summary

1. Claims are examined to determine whether benefits are due to patients according to the policy and whether the services the patient received were medically necessary. At times, additional clinical information is required to process a claim.

2. The five steps for processing RAs are: (a) match the claim control number, patient's name, and date of service with the payer's payments; (b) check the patient data, plan, and listed procedures against the claim; (c) compare the payment for each procedure with the expected amount; (d) read the carrier's explanations for unpaid, reduced, or denied claims and decide if a resubmission or appeal is warranted; and (e) determine the amounts of any write-offs that must be entered as adjustments in the patient's account, and note the balance due from the patient.

3. Health plans may reduce or deny claims because the patient is not currently enrolled or up-to-date with required premiums, the services are not covered by the patient's policy or are deemed not medically necessary, or the linkage between diagnoses and procedures does not satisfy the payer. The physician or the patient may decide to appeal the payer's determination. An appeal is the process of reviewing benefit reimbursement questions. If an appeal does not resolve a reimbursement issue, a peer review by an unbiased group of physicians may be requested. Appeals may also be resolved by asking the state insurance commissioner to make a ruling on a dispute.

4. After an office visit, the new charges are entered into the patient's account in the billing program. If the physician is not filing a claim for the patient, the patient is charged for the services, often paying at the end of the visit. If the physician is filing a claim, the patient pays a copayment if required at the time of service and then is billed for the balance due after the insurance carrier's payment is recorded. After patient bills are sent, the collections process is used to collect overdue payments.

5. Often, patients do not understand insurance billing issues. The medical insurance specialist should offer to help patients resolve them. When explaining an insurance issue to a patient, speech should be slow and calm, and simple language should be used. Information may need to be explained more than once.

Check Your Understanding

Part 1. Choose the best answer.

c **1.** It has been thirty days since a claim was filed, and no response has arrived from the carrier. The best thing to do is:
   a. wait another ten days
   b. inform the physician
   c. contact the health plan

b **2.** A mistake on a claim already paid is discovered. The medical insurance specialist should:
   a. write off the unpaid amount
   b. rebill according to the payer's instructions
   c. send the patient a bill

c **3.** A claim was denied. Which of the following was not the reason?
   a. preexisting condition
   b. coverage cancellation
   c. vacationing carrier representative

a **4.** A letter from the carrier states that not enough information was submitted to process a claim. The medical insurance specialist should:
   a. make sure all the necessary information is provided
   b. send the letter to the patient
   c. make a note in the patient's record to rebill in thirty days

c **5.** The RA summarizes payments for:
   a. a single patient
   b. a single claim
   c. multiple patients and claims

c **6.** Collections are done on bills that are classified as:
   a. current
   b. written off
   c. past due

b **7.** Which report is used by billers to follow up on late claims from health plans?
   a. patient aging
   b. insurance aging
   c. patient ledger

c **8.** The abbreviation EFT means
   a. electric forwarding transmission
   b. eventual follow-up of transfer
   c. electronic funds transfer

b **9.** Uncollectible accounts are:
   a. reported to health plans
   b. written off
   c. reported to CMS

Part 2. Calculate the balances due from the four patients listed in Figure 7-2:

A. Angelo Daiute

B. Brian Daiute

C. Mary F. Daiute

D. Rosemary B. Daiute

Part 3. Determine the amount due from the patient of a PAR physician based on the following information from the RA, explaining your reasoning.

Charges:	$25.00
Disallowed:	$3.42
Allowed Charge:	$21.58
Deductible:	0
Coinsurance:	$10.00
Amount Due from Carrier:	$11.58
Additional Amount Due from Patient:	$ _10.00_

21.58
−11.58
10.00

Blue Cross and Blue Shield

Objectives

After completing this chapter, you will be able to define the key terms and:

1. Discuss the history and structure of the Blue Cross and Blue Shield organization.
2. Describe four key features of Blue Cross and Blue Shield member plans.
3. Compare the responsibilities of physicians who do and do not participate in Blue Cross and Blue Shield member plans.
4. Explain the BlueCard Program.
5. Describe important data to obtain from a subscriber's Blue Cross and Blue Shield card.
6. State two reasons to complete claim forms within established time limits.

Key Terms

BlueCard Program
BlueCard Worldwide
Blue Cross
Blue Cross and Blue Shield
  Association (BCBS)

Blue Shield
certificate
Federal Employee Health
  Benefits (FEHB) plan
home plan

host plan
member plan
nationwide plan
out-of-area program

Why This Chapter Is Important to You

The information in this chapter will enable you to:

- Learn about an important insurance carrier that you will work with frequently as a medical insurance specialist
- Learn rules for processing claims for the Blue Cross and Blue Shield BlueCard Program and BlueCard Worldwide program
- Become familiar with terms that apply to Blue Cross and Blue Shield coverage

What Do You Think?

Blue Cross and Blue Shield is a national association with affiliated plans in each state. If a new patient presents a Blue Cross and Blue Shield card, how does the medical insurance specialist verify insurance coverage?

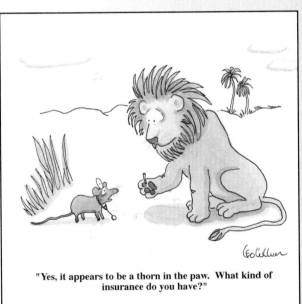

"Yes, it appears to be a thorn in the paw. What kind of insurance do you have?"

The Blue Cross and Blue Shield Association (BCBS) is a group of individual, independently licensed local companies. The association itself is not an insurance provider. Instead, it licenses the Blue Cross and Blue Shield brands and membership standards to the individual health coverage plans. Locally owned Blue Cross and Blue Shield companies that provide this coverage are known as member plans.

The Blue Cross and Blue Shield Association was developed from two kinds of health care programs: Blue Cross, which covered hospital services, and Blue Shield, which covered physician services. Today, Blue Cross has expanded its coverage from inpatient care to include benefits for outpatient and home care services, as well as other kinds of institutional care. Blue Shield plans, in addition to physician services, now offer specialty plans for dental, vision, mental health, prescription, and hearing services and other outpatient benefits. These plans may be added to an existing BCBS plan, or they may be purchased as stand-alone plans.

The first Blue Cross plan was founded in 1929 at Baylor University in Dallas, Texas. Teachers there agreed to pay $6 per year in exchange for twenty-one days of care at the university hospital, should the need arise. The first Blue Shield plan, founded in 1939 to provide physician services, was known as the California Physicians' Service. Its membership was restricted to individuals who earned less than $3,000 per year. The first members paid a monthly premium of $1.70.

Soon after these plans began, additional employee groups and health care providers joined, and similar programs were started in other communities. Today, most BCBS plans operate as joint corporations, but some remain separate organizations. They all belong to the Blue Cross and Blue Shield Association. There are over forty-two independent plans with a total enrollment of nearly 89 million people. About one-half of the members are in preferred provider organizations (PPOs), one-quarter in indemnity plans, and another 20 percent in health maintenance organizations (HMOs).

The Blue Cross and Blue Shield Association represents member plans in matters of national scope; encourages cost-containment practices; develops evaluation methods for new technology; provides research, marketing, and actuarial services; coordinates public relations, advertising, public education, and professional relations programs; and administers membership standards. In addition, the association coordinates the claim process for nationwide plans, which are large membership accounts with offices located throughout the country. It also administers Medicare and other federal and state health programs.

> **HIPAA Tip**
>
> For BCBS claims, enter the subscriber's group number as it appears on the membership card. When entering the name of the member plan, be sure to include the state or the geographic area, such as Blue Cross and Blue Shield of Illinois, if this is part of the plan name.

FEDERAL EMPLOYEE HEALTH BENEFITS PLAN

Employees of the federal government may select the BCBS Federal Employee Health Benefits (FEHB) plan as their health insurance plan. The FEHB plan, which began in 1960, is the largest privately underwritten health insurance contract in the world. Federal employees enroll in a fee-for-service program that operates as a PPO. Members may enroll in a Standard Option plan or a Basic Option plan. Under the Standard Option plan, members may choose to receive treatment from a physician within the PPO network (the most cost-effective option) or outside the network (at a higher cost). Under the Basic Option plan, members must use PPO providers in order to receive benefits. (Some exceptions apply, such as for emergency care.) Both plans require copayments and coinsurance. Under Standard Option, members must also pay applicable deductibles.

KEY FEATURES OF BLUE CROSS AND BLUE SHIELD PLANS

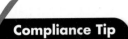
Compliance Tip

BCBS member plans offer subscribers a variety of benefit packages that range from fee-for-service to managed care plans. Many plans require preauthorization and second opinions. Because each subscriber's package may have different rules, and because the details of each plan are negotiated regularly, it is important to get complete and up-to-date information from the patient's local member plan to ensure prompt payment of health care claims.

BCBS member plans cover their members' health care costs in much the same way as commercial insurance companies do for their policyholders. Some different terms, however, are used. A patient enrolled in a BCBS plan, referred to as a subscriber, is issued a certificate, not a policy. This certificate lists the benefits and responsibilities of the plan. A subscriber receives coverage directly from a BCBS member plan, through a small or large private employer, or through the federal government or a state government.

Because the BCBS Association was founded by state hospital associations and medical societies in the 1930s to provide low-cost, basic insurance, many BCBS member plans still operate as charitable, or nonprofit, corporations. Unlike commercial insurers that distribute profits to stockholders, these BCBS plans pay out about ninety cents of every premium dollar as benefits to subscribers. The remaining 10 percent of their income goes for operating expenses and reserves. Reserves are required by law in case operating expenses or abnormally high claims exceed expectations. BCBS member plans that operate as nonprofit organizations cannot raise rates without approval from state departments of insurance. The process often includes a public hearing. Note, however, that some states require all carriers to get approval for rate increases.

In 1994, the BCBS Association gave permission for member companies to be owned by investors. Since then, some member companies have become investor-owned and for-profit. For example, in 2003 Anthem, Inc., a health care company that owned BCBS plans in nine states (Indiana, Kentucky, Ohio, Connecticut, New Hampshire, Colorado, Nevada, Maine, and Virginia) merged with Wellpoint Health Networks, Inc., which owned BCBS plans in four states (California, Georgia, Missouri, and Wisconsin). This merger created an investor-owned for-profit company that owns BCBS plans in thirteen states.

BCBS member plans often accept subscribers whom other carriers will not cover. Many small groups and individuals who may not be able to get coverage elsewhere can join Blue Cross and Blue Shield. Some member plans offer coverage regardless of medical condition during special enrollment periods. This widespread availability means that more people have medical insurance, thus reducing the number of bad debts and charity cases physicians and other health care providers absorb.

Health care providers can sign participation contracts with BCBS member plans. Providers who sign these contracts agree to submit all claims on behalf of patients and to accept the BCBS allowed amounts as payment in full for covered services. Most plans determine payment amounts to participating providers based on the standard methods of establishing fee schedules. Participating providers may not engage in balance billing. Payment is made directly to all participating providers.

Participating providers may also choose to contract with BCBS's Preferred Provider Network (PPN). A PPN contract requires physicians to adhere to network regulations, including providing quality service, properly utilizing services and resources, and containing the cost of services. In addition, PPN members agree to accept fees that are slightly lower than those for participating providers who are not PPN members. There are several advantages to PPN membership: physicians are notified when new groups enroll in the PPN, and those groups are given a physician directory that lists all members.

At times, a patient may see a physician who is not a plan participant. When the physician is a nonparticipating (nonPAR) provider, payment is made directly to the patient, even if the nonparticipating provider files the claim. A nonparticipating provider can collect the entire fee from a member patient, even if the fee exceeds plan payment levels.

FILING CLAIMS FOR SPECIAL CASES AND NATIONAL GROUPS

The Blue Cross and Blue Shield Association administers the BlueCard Program, which is an out-of-area program that allows for reciprocal coverage while a subscriber is away from the local area. An out-of-area program covers specific services for a member who receives care at a host plan elsewhere. The home plan, the plan that the subscriber contracts with, usually keeps all information on membership and claims for the subscriber.

The BlueCard Program links the participating health care providers and the independent BCBS member plans across the United States through a single electronic network for claims processing and reimbursement. The program makes sure that subscribers have health care services while they are traveling or living in another member plan's service area. The subscribers have the same benefits as in their plan and access to BlueCard providers.

When an out-of-area BCBS membership card is presented to a participating provider, the provider verifies the membership and coverage by contacting BlueCard Eligibility. The provider then files the claim with the local host plan, which sends the claim to the subscriber's home plan. The subscriber's home plan processes it and sends the approved claim back to the local host plan, which pays the provider. The home plan also sends the subscriber an explanation of benefits.

For example, Emma Block, a New York resident and a member of a New York BCBS member plan, has surgery in Kansas City to have her gallbladder removed. Through the BlueCard Program, a Kansas City participating physician will perform the surgery and bill Blue Cross and Blue Shield of Kansas City. The physician will receive reimbursement according to the Kansas City plan's payment method.

BLUECARD WORLDWIDE

The BlueCard Program also contains an international component, called BlueCard Worldwide. This plan allows BCBS plan members traveling or living abroad to receive the benefits they would receive at home. As with the domestic BlueCard program, BlueCard Worldwide links a network of participating BCBS health care providers and hospitals outside the United States with the independent BCBS member plans in the United States in an attempt to provide the same level of coverage abroad that members receive at home and to coordinate claims processing and reimbursement.

MEMBERSHIP CARD INFORMATION

A Blue Cross and Blue Shield plan membership card contains vital information needed to file claims for member patients. The front and back of the card should be photocopied and placed in the patient's medical record for easy reference. The copy of this card should be updated annually or whenever the patient receives a new card.

In addition to the subscriber's name, most BCBS cards have the following information: plan name; type of plan; subscriber identification number (usually the subscriber's Social Security number with a three-letter alpha prefix); effective date of coverage; BCBS plan codes and coverage codes; participation in a reciprocity plan with other BCBS plans; copayments, coinsurance, and deductible amounts; information about additional coverage, such as prescription medication or mental-health care; information about preauthorization requirements; claims submission address; and contact phone numbers. Figure 8-1 shows the front and back of a typical card.

MEDICAL PROGRAM:
EMERGENCY ROOM COPAY $50.00
COINSURANCE   30%
SINGLE DEDUCTIBLE $2500.00
FAMILY DEDUCTIBLE $5000.00

To obtain your discounted prescription, please present this card to the Pharmacist.

CLAIMS SUBMISSION: MENTAL HEALTH/SUBSTANCE ABUSE
HORIZON BCBSNJ   MAGELLAN BEHAVIORAL HEALTH
PO BOX 1609   199 POMEROY ROAD
NEWARK, NEW JERSEY 07101-1609   PARSIPPANY, NEW JERSEY 07054-2820

CUSTOMER SERVICE 1-800-355-BLUE

ATTENTION MEMBERS & PROVIDERS:

SPECIAL PROGRAMS INCLUDE: PRE-ADMISSION REVIEW
& MANDATORY SECOND SURGICAL OPINION

Pre-Admission Review is required prior to all inpatient admissions. Emergency admissions require notification within 48 hours. In a potentially life threatening situation, call "911" or your local emergency number. The emergency response team not your insurance carrier is responsible for response times and failures to respond. A second opinion is required for certain procedures. Failure to comply will result in reduced benefits. For mental health or substance abuse, please call Magellan Behavioral Health's confidential, 24 hour, toll free help line at 1-800-626-2212.

Horizon.
Horizon Blue Cross Blue Shield
of New Jersey
An Independent Licensee of the Blue Cross and Blue Shield Association

NAME   **D SANDS**
ID NUMBER   **NSD155685526**
COVERAGE CODE   B1060
TYPE   SINGLE
EFFECTIVE DATE 06/01/2008   **HORIZON TRADITIONAL**
BC/BS PLAN CODES 280/780   **PLAN C**
RXBIN   004336
RXPCN   HZRX ISSUER(80840)   AdvancePCS
                                      Prescription Benefit Services

SPECIAL PROGRAMS CONTACT: 1-800-624-1294

PRESCRIPTION CLAIMS: AdvancePCS
                     P.O. Box 853901
                     Richardson, TX 75085-3901

Figure 8-1 Sample of BCBS Identification Card

The BCBS plan identification cards for FEHB subscribers include the words "Government-wide Service Benefit Plan" and also specify the level of the plan. Individuals enrolled in low-option plans pay higher deductibles and copayments than individuals in high-option plans. The coverage of the plans is similar.

FILING DEADLINES

Explore the Internet

Visit the Web site for the national Blue Cross and Blue Shield Association at http://www.bcbs.com. Enter your ZIP code, and look up information about the Blue Cross and Blue Shield affiliate for the state in which you live. What types of plans are offered?

As a matter of routine, most medical offices file insurance claims on a regular basis, usually within a thirty-day billing cycle. Timely filing means prompt reimbursement, especially for BCBS claims. However, that is not the only reason for efficient insurance claims procedures.

BCBS's contracts with participating providers specify timely filing guidelines, which are various time limits for filing claims. Failure to submit claims to the member plan within the contracted time frame results in refusal to pay. If this happens, the provider cannot bill the subscriber either; the physician cannot collect fees for these services at all. Although exceptions can be made for special circumstances, every effort should be made to meet the contract's filing deadlines.

Professional Focus

Blue Cross and Blue Shield

In this first decade of this century, the Blue Cross and Blue Shield Association's member plans insure more than 89 million—or one in four—U.S. citizens. BCBS member plans provide a variety of health care plans, including health maintenance organizations (HMOs), preferred provider organizations (PPOs), point-of-service (POS) programs, and fee-for-service coverage. They are the nation's largest provider of managed care services.

Chapter Summary

1. The Blue Cross and Blue Shield Association is a national group of local companies that offer prepaid coverage for health care. Blue Cross was founded in 1929 to cover hospital care. Blue Shield was founded in 1939 to cover physician services. Today, most local Blue Cross and Blue Shield member plans operate as joint corporations. The plans belong to the national Blue Cross and Blue Shield Association.

2. Four features of Blue Cross and Blue Shield member plans are that (a) they issue certificates to subscribers; (b) many are nonprofit, or charitable, organizations that cannot raise rates without state approval; (c) they offer unique contractual relationships with health care providers; and (d) they are widely available to individuals and small groups.

3. Participating providers must file all claims for their patients and must accept the BCBS fee schedule. Nonparticipating providers do not file claims directly with the BCBS plan; the patient pays the provider and then files a claim with the plan. NonPARs can charge their usual fees to BCBS patients.

4. The BlueCard Program allows host plans to process claims for services performed in their communities for patients covered by BCBS home plans in other areas.

5. The BlueCard Worldwide program allows plan members to receive the same level of coverage abroad that they would receive at home.

6. The information listed on a BCBS subscriber's identification card usually includes plan name; type of plan; subscriber identification number; effective date of coverage; BCBS plan codes and coverage codes; participation in a reciprocity plan with other BCBS plans; copayments, coinsurance, and deductible amounts; additional coverage; preauthorization requirements; claims submission address; and contact information.

7. Two reasons to complete BCBS claim forms within timely filing guidelines are to ensure prompt payment and to prevent the member plan from refusing to honor the claim for payment.

Check Your Understanding

Part 1. In the space provided, write the word or phrase that best completes each sentence.

1. _____ was first established to cover physician services.

2. Blue Cross and Blue Shield member plans operate as _____ corporations.

3. The _____ pays the PAR provider under the BlueCard Program.

4. _____ was established to cover hospital expenses.

5. The _____ covers Blue Cross and Blue Shield plan subscribers who travel nationally.

6. The Blue Cross and Blue Shield Association does not provide _____.

7. Large Blue Cross and Blue Shield membership accounts with offices throughout the country are called _____.

8. Another name for a Blue Cross and Blue Shield plan member is a(n) _____.

9. The _____ covers Blue Cross and Blue Shield plan subscribers who travel abroad.

10. The BCBS _____ is a health insurance plan for employees of the federal government.

Part 2. Supply the answers to the following two cases.

A.
Physician Information:
Name: Mary Kant, MD
NPI: 5678901234
Blue Cross and Blue Shield Provider ID Number: 21-8554-56

Patient Information Form:
Name: William D. Degracia (New Patient)
Age: 24
Sex: Male
Birth Date: October 11, 1984
Marital Status: Single
Employer: Cone Plumbing and Air Conditioning
Insurance Carrier: Anthem Blue Cross and Blue Shield
Insured's ID Number: 088-09-7675
Insured's Group Number: G68063
Insured's Plan Name: BlueCare Plus Direct (HMO)

Patient's Encounter Form:
Date: 6-25-2008
T-99   BP 127/83
CC: Redness and swelling, right big toe.
Dx: Paronychia, right big toe.
Rx: Bacitracin to be applied.

List of Fees for Service:

Charges: Office visit, ten-minute exam, problem-focused, straightforward decision making, $45; office visit copayment charge, $20

Amount collected: $20, office visit copayment

Supply the following data elements:

Billing Provider _____

Billing Provider's Primary Identifier _____

Billing Provider's Secondary Identifier _____

Subscriber/Patient _____

Subscriber's Primary Identifier _____

Claim Filing Indicator Code _____

Payer Name/ID _____

Place of Service Code _____

Diagnosis Codes _____

Total Charge _____

Amount Collected _____

Service Line Information

Date of Service _____

Procedure Code/Charge _____

Diagnosis _____

Date of Service _____

Procedure Code/Charge _____

Diagnosis _____

B.

Physician Information:
Name: Michael A. Hardinsky, MD
NPI: 6789012345
Blue Cross and Blue Shield Provider ID Number: 0003480000-00

Patient Information Form:
Name: Susan A. Beeme (Established Patient)
Sex: Female
Birth Date: February 14, 1993
Responsible Person: Jennifer Beeme (mother)
Birth Date: May 12, 1963
Marital Status: Divorced
Employer: Runnymeade Court Realty
Insurance Carrier: Anthem Blue Cross and Blue Shield
Insured's ID Number: 24536574-02
Insured's Group Number: 00041
Insured's Plan Name: Blue Traditional (indemnity plan)

Patient Encounter Form:
Date: 6-25-2008
T-99   BP 127/83
CC: Patient's diabetes first diagnosed April 12, 2003; presents for diabetes recheck; lab workup shows acceptable range from about 78 to mid-100s with an occasional number over 200. Overall control is good.
Dx: Diabetes Mellitus, type II.

List of Fees for Service:
Office visit with problem-focused history and examination; straightforward decision making $65
Lab: Urinalysis by dip stick ($6); quantitative glucose analysis, blood ($9)
Amount collected: 20% copayment, $16.00

Supply the following data elements:

Billing Provider _____

Billing Provider's Primary Identifier _____

Billing Provider's Secondary Identifier _____

Subscriber _____

Patient _____

Relationship _____

Subscriber's Primary Identifier _____

Claim Filing Indicator Code _____

Payer Name/ID _____

Place of Service Code _____

Diagnosis Codes _____

Total Charge _____

Amount Collected _____

Service Line Information

Date of Service _____

Procedure Code/Charge _____

Diagnosis _____

Date of Service _____

Procedure Code/Charge _____

Diagnosis _____

Date of Service _____

Procedure Code/Charge _____

Diagnosis _____

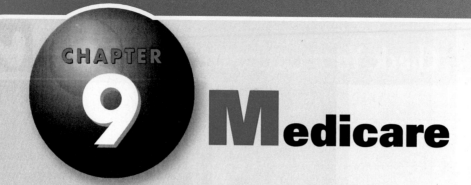

CHAPTER 9 Medicare

Objectives

After completing this chapter, you will be able to define the key terms and:

1. Identify two parts of Medicare coverage.
2. Discuss the fees that Medicare participating and nonparticipating physicians are allowed to charge.
3. Explain the difference between an excluded service and a medically unnecessary service.
4. Name four situations in which Medicare is the secondary payer.

Key Terms

advance beneficiary notice (ABN)
crossover claims
diagnosis-related groups (DRGs)
fiscal intermediary
Health Savings Account
hospice
limiting charge
Medicare

Medicare Advantage
Medicare beneficiary
Medicare Fee Schedule (MFS)
Medicare Modernization Act (MMA)
Medicare Part A
Medicare Part B
Medicare Remittance Notice (MRN)

Medicare Summary Notice (MSN)
Medigap insurance
Medi-Medi
Notice of Exclusions from Medicare Benefits (NEMB)
Original Medicare Plan
primary payer
secondary payer

Why This Chapter Is Important to You

The information in this chapter will enable you to:

- Become familiar with the federal health insurance plan for older Americans and some people with disabilities
- Explain Medicare coverage to patients
- File Medicare claims correctly

What Do You Think?

Two factors, demographics and politics, are large influences on Medicare. First, the portion of the country's population that is elderly and eligible for Medicare is increasing rapidly. The baby boom generation (people born between 1946 and 1964) will reach retirement age between 2010 and 2030. The 65 million Americans over sixty-five will make up 21 percent of the population. Over the past forty years, the number of people over eighty-five has grown at a much faster rate than the overall population. At the start of this century, 1.6 percent of the population—more than 4 million people—is over eighty-five years of age.

Second, with more people on Medicare's rolls and with new legislation offering prescription drug benefits for the first time, the costs of the program add up to a significant share of the federal budget. To offset these costs, CMS, which runs Medicare, has put a number of cost controls and billing regulations in place.

Since CMS mandates that a physician who treats a Medicare patient must also complete the claim for the patient, medical insurance specialists often handle many Medicare claims. What resources can be used to stay up to date about changes in this important system?

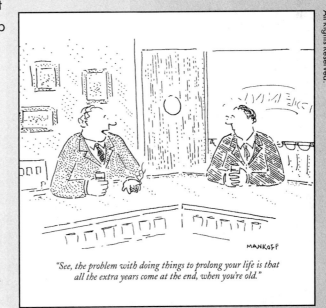

"See, the problem with doing things to prolong your life is that all the extra years come at the end, when you're old."

MEDICARE OVERVIEW

The federal health insurance program for people who are sixty-five or older is known as Medicare. Medicare also provides benefits to people with some disabilities and end-stage renal disease (ESRD), which is permanent kidney failure. A person covered by Medicare is called a Medicare beneficiary. Some beneficiaries qualify through the Social Security Administration. Others are eligible through the Railroad Retirement System. Medicare has two parts, one for care given by institutions and the other for services by physicians.

The federal government does not pay Medicare claims directly. Instead, it contracts with insurance organizations to process claims on its behalf. Insurance companies that process claims for hospitals, skilled nursing facilities, intermediate care facilities, long-term care facilities, and home health care agencies are known as fiscal intermediaries. Insurance companies that process claims for physicians, providers, and suppliers are referred to as carriers.

Medicare Part A

Medicare Part A helps pay for inpatient hospital services, care in a skilled nursing facility, home health care, and hospice care. A hospice is a public or private organization that provides services for terminally ill patients and their families. Hospice care extends beyond medical services to include psychological and spiritual care.

Fees paid by Medicare Part A for inpatient hospital services are based on diagnosis-related groups (DRGs). Under this system, groups of hospital cases across the country have been analyzed to arrive at the fixed fees Medicare pays for hospital services. The DRG number for the payment is assigned based on the principal diagnosis.

Those who are eligible for Social Security benefits are automatically enrolled in Medicare Part A. They do not have to pay insurance premiums. Although people age sixty-five or older who do not qualify for Social Security benefits have the option of enrolling in Part A, they must pay premiums to get benefits.

Medicare Part B

Medicare Part B helps pay for physician services, outpatient hospital services, durable medical equipment, and other services and supplies. All Medicare providers must file claims on behalf of patients at no cost to the patients. Medical office insurance specialists file claims under Part B for physician services, even if the services are performed in a hospital setting. They do not usually file claims for Part A benefits.

Part B coverage is optional. Everyone who is eligible for Part A may choose to enroll in Part B by paying monthly premiums (usually deducted automatically from Social Security retirement benefit payments). Therefore, the medical insurance specialist should check the patient's Medicare identification card for coverage information each visit, since coverage may be renewed monthly in some states and might expire between office visits.

Medicare Insurance Card

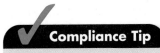

Compliance Tip

The Medicare Prescription Drug, Improvement, and Modernization Act of 2003, called the **Medicare Modernization Act (MMA)**, includes a number of changes that will roll out over a period of years, including a prescription drug benefit. Medical insurance specialists must keep up to date with changes affecting their practices' patients for correct billing and reimbursement.

Each Medicare enrollee receives a health insurance card (see Figure 9-1). This card lists the beneficiary's name, sex, and Medicare number, and the effective dates for Part A and Part B coverage. The Medicare number is assigned by the Centers for Medicare and Medicaid Services (CMS) and usually consists of the Social Security number followed by a numeric or alphanumeric ending. The letter at the end provides additional information about the patient. For example, A stands for wage earner, B for spouse's number, and D for widow/er.

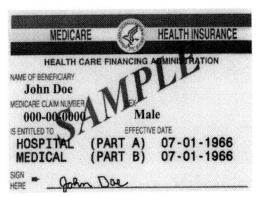

Figure 9-1 Sample Medicare Patient Identification Card

Medicare Part B Plans

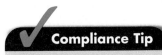

Compliance Tip

The Original Medicare Plan is administered by the Center for Medicare Management, a department of CMS.

Medicare beneficiaries can choose from among a number of insurance plans. Medicare beneficiaries who enroll in the Medicare fee-for-service plan (referred to by Medicare as the Original Medicare Plan) can choose any licensed physician certified by Medicare. They must pay the premium, the coinsurance (which is 20 percent), and the annual deductible specified each year by the Medicare law, which is voted on by Congress. How much of a patient's medical bills has been applied to the annual deductible is shown on the Medicare Remittance Notice (MRN) that the office receives and also on the Medicare Summary Notice (MSN) the patient receives. Each time a beneficiary receives services, a fee is billable. Most offices bill the patient for any balance due after the MRN is received, rather than at the time of the appointment.

Medicare also offers a group of plans called Medicare Advantage (formerly Medicare+Choice). Beneficiaries can choose to enroll in one of these types of plans, instead of the Original Medicare Plan:

- Medicare managed care plans
- Medicare preferred provider organization plans (PPOs)
- Medicare private fee-for-service plans
- Health Savings Accounts

Medicare Managed Care Plans

Some beneficiaries choose to join managed care plans such as HMOs for Part B coverage. Most managed care plans charge monthly premiums and small copayments for office visits, but not deductibles. Medicare managed

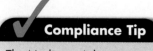
care plans, like other managed care plans, often require patients to use a specific network of physicians, hospitals, and facilities. Some plans offer patients the option of seeing providers outside the network for a higher fee. On the other hand, they offer coverage for services not reimbursed in fee-for-service plans, such as routine physical examinations or additional days in the hospital.

Managed care plans offer beneficiaries a number of advantages:

- Low copayment when receiving treatment
- Minimal paperwork
- Coverage for additional services
- No need for a supplemental Medigap policy (see below)

Disadvantages of Medicare managed care plans include the following:

- Physician choices limited to those in the particular plan
- Typically need to obtain prior approval from the primary care physician (PCP) before seeing a specialist, undergoing elective surgery, and receiving other services

Preferred Provider Organization (PPO)

In the Medicare preferred provider organization plan (PPO), patients are given a financial incentive to use doctors within a network, but they may choose to go outside the network. Visits outside the network incur additional costs, which may include a higher copayment or higher coinsurance. A PPO contracts with a certain group of providers to offer health care services to patients. Unlike HMOs, many PPOs do not require patients to select a PCP.

Private Fee-for-Service (PFFS)

Under a private fee-for-service plan, patients receive services from the provider or facility of their choosing, as long as Medicare has approved the provider or facility. The plan is operated by a private insurance company that contracts with Medicare to provide services to beneficiaries. The plan sets its own rates for services, and physicians are allowed to bill patients the amount of the charge not covered by the plan, as long as it does not exceed 15 percent. A copayment may or may not be required. Under a private fee-for-service plan, patients may pay rates that are higher or lower than the rates on the Medicare Fee Schedule, but they cannot be charged for balance billing.

Health Savings Accounts

The Medicare Modernization Act creates a plan for Medicare called a Health Savings Account. Similar to private medical savings accounts, this plan combines a high-deductible fee-for-service plan with a tax-exempt trust to pay for qualified medical expenses. The deductible must be at least $1,000 a year for individuals and $2,000 for couples.

MEDICARE CHARGES

The Medicare Fee Schedule (MFS) is the basis for payments for all Original Medicare Plan services. This national system is based on the Resource-Based Relative Value Scale (RBRVS) system using cost factors that represent the physician's time and how much it costs to run a practice (see Chapter 5).

Participation

Annually, physicians choose whether they want to participate in the Medicare program. Participating physicians agree to accept assignment for all Medicare claims and to accept Medicare's allowed charge according to the Medicare Fee Schedule as payment in full for services. A PAR physician may bill the patient for coinsurance and deductibles but may not collect amounts higher than the Medicare amount allowed by the fee schedule. Medicare is responsible for paying 80 percent of this allowed charge (after patients have met their annual deductibles). Patients are responsible for the other 20 percent. The physician may bill the patient for services not covered by Medicare.

Example

A Medicare PAR provider has a usual charge of $200 for a diagnostic flexible sigmoidoscopy (CPT 45330), and the Medicare-allowed charge is $84. The provider must write off the difference between the two charges. The patient is responsible for 20 percent of the allowed charge, not of the provider's usual charge:

Provider's usual fee:	$200.00
Medicare allowed charge:	$ 84.00
Medicare pays 80 percent	$ 67.20
Patient pays 20 percent	$ 16.80

The total the provider can collect is $84. The provider must write off the difference between the usual fee and the allowed charge, $116.

Nonparticipation

Nonparticipating physicians decide whether to accept assignment on a claim-by-claim basis. Providers who elect not to participate in the Medicare program but who accept assignment on a claim are paid 5 percent less for their services than PAR providers. For example, if the Medicare-allowed amount for a service is $100, the PAR provider receives $80 (80 percent of $100), and the nonPAR provider receives $76 ($80 minus 5 percent). Non-PAR providers who do not accept assignment are subject to Medicare's charge limits. They may not charge a Medicare patient more than 115 percent of the amount listed in the Medicare nonparticipating fee schedule. This amount—115 percent of the fee listed in the nonPAR MFS—is called the limiting charge.

For a nonassigned claim, the provider can collect the full payment of the limiting charge from the patient at the time of the visit. The claim is then submitted to Medicare. If approved, Medicare will pay 80 percent of the allowed amount on the nonPAR fee schedule—not the limiting amount. Medicare sends this payment directly to the patient, since the physician has already been paid.

Example

The following example illustrates the different fee structures for PARs, nonPARs who accept assignment, and nonPARs who do not accept assignment.

Participating Provider

Physician's standard fee	$120.00
Medicare fee	$60.00
Medicare pays 80% ($60.00 × 80%)	$48.00
Patient or supplemental plan pays 20% ($60.00 × 20%)	$12.00
Provider adjustment (write-off) ($120.00 – $60.00)	$60.00

Nonparticipating Provider (Accepts Assignment)

Physician's standard fee	$120.00
Medicare nonPAR fee ($60.00 – 5%)	$57.00
Medicare pays 80% ($57.00 × 80%)	$45.60
Patient or supplemental plan pays 20% ($57.00 × 20%)	$11.40
Provider adjustment (write-off) ($120.00 – $57.00)	$63.00

Nonparticipating Provider (Does Not Accept Assignment)

Physician's standard fee	$120.00
Medicare nonPAR fee ($60.00 – 5%)	$57.00
Limiting charge (115% × 57.00)	$65.55
Patient billed	$65.55
Medicare pays patient (80% × 65.55)	$52.44
Total provider can collect	$65.55
Patient out-of-pocket expense ($65.55 – $52.44)	$13.11

> **✓ Compliance Tip**
>
> Physicians must accept assignment for clinical diagnostic laboratory services (generally, procedures with CPT codes in the 80000s). The physician may not bill Medicare patients for these services. If the physician does not accept Medicare assignment for them, the right to bill the patient is forfeited. The physician may accept assignment for laboratory services only, and refuse to accept assignment for other services. In this case, two separate claims may be filed. One claim accepts assignment for laboratory services, and the other refuses assignment for other services.

FILING MEDICARE CLAIMS

Physicians who treat Medicare beneficiaries must file claims for their patients even if they do not participate and do not accept assignment on the claims. CMS mandates electronic transmission of Medicare claims using the HIPAA 837 format, except for very small practices and for those that never send any kind of electronic health care transactions.

Filing Medicare claims is similar to filing claims for other plans, with one main exception. Procedure codes for Medicare claims come from the Healthcare Common Procedure Coding System (HCPCS). As covered in Chapter 4, this coding system is made up of CPT codes and national codes. As with CPT codes, modifiers may be used with HCPCS codes. These modifiers are different from CPT modifiers. The medical insurance specialist must be careful to use CPT modifiers with CPT codes and HCPCS modifiers with HCPCS codes.

Medicare's Correct Coding Initiative

Medicare's National Correct Coding Council develops correct coding guidelines in order to control improper procedural coding in Part B claims. This council issues policies, called the Correct Coding Initiative (CCI), to correct two types of errors: (1) unintentional coding errors resulting from a misunderstanding of coding, and (2) intentionally incorrect coding done to increase payments. CCI guidelines are part of the automatic edits for electronic claims.

Since CCI has been in place, Medicare claim rejections have multiplied. The most common cause for rejection is unbundling, a term for breaking out and reporting procedures separately that should be reported under a single code for an entire procedure. Under CCI, if the services are provided to a beneficiary on a single day and by a single physician, the coder must double-check for any bundled codes (see Chapter 4) that may apply. Entering the correct codes on claims saves the medical office time and money in resubmitting rejected claims.

Excluded Services and Not Medically Necessary Services

Medicare does not provide coverage for certain services and procedures. Claims will be denied when the service provided is excluded by Medicare, or because the service was not reasonable and necessary for the specific patient.

Excluded Services

Excluded services are those that are not covered under any circumstances, such as routine physical examinations and many screening tests. These services change from year to year. While not required, it is good practice to provide patients with written notification that Medicare does not pay for the service before providing it and an estimate of how much they may have to pay. The CMS form Notice of Exclusions from Medicare Benefits (NEMB) may be used (see Figure 9.2 on page 154), or providers may design their own NEMBs based on the particular services they offer.

Medically Unnecessary Services

Services that the Medicare program does not consider generally medically necessary are not covered unless certain conditions are met, such as the relation of the procedure, treatment, or service to the diagnoses. For example, a vitamin B12 injection is a covered service only for patients with certain diagnoses, such as pernicious anemia. To be considered medically necessary, a treatment must be:

- Appropriate for the symptoms or diagnoses of the illness or injury
- Not elective
- Not an experimental or investigational procedure
- An essential treatment, not one performed for the patient's convenience
- Delivered at the most appropriate level that can safely and effectively be administered to the patient

Several common categories of medical necessity denials include:

- Improper Linkage Between the Diagnosis and the Service—The diagnosis does not justify the procedures performed. The denial may result from a clerical error (for example, a fifth digit was missing from an ICD-9-CM code). In many of these instances, the claim can be corrected and will eventually be paid. In other situations, the diagnosis is not specific enough to justify the treatment.

NOTICE OF EXCLUSIONS FROM MEDICARE BENEFITS (NEMB)
There are items and services for which Medicare will not pay.

- Medicare does **not** pay for all of your health care costs. Medicare only pays for covered benefits. **Some items and services are not Medicare benefits and Medicare will not pay for them.**
- When you receive an item or service that is not a Medicare benefit, **you are responsible to pay for it,** personally or through any other insurance that you may have.

The purpose of this notice is to help you make an informed choice about whether or not you want to receive these items or services, knowing that you will have to pay for them yourself. **Before you make a decision, you should read this entire notice carefully.**

Ask us to explain, if you don't understand why Medicare won't pay.

Ask us how much these items or services will cost you (**Estimated Cost: $_____**).

Medicare will not pay for: _____

_____;

- ❑ **1. Because it does not meet the definition of any Medicare benefit.**

- ❑ **2. Because of the following exclusion * from Medicare benefits:**

❑ Personal comfort items.	❑ Routine physicals and most tests for screening.
❑ Most shots (vaccinations).	❑ Routine eye care, eyeglasses and examinations.
❑ Hearing aids and hearing examinations.	❑ Cosmetic surgery.
❑ Most outpatient prescription drugs.	❑ Dental care and dentures (in most cases).
❑ Orthopedic shoes and foot supports (orthotics).	❑ Routine foot care and flat foot care.
❑ Health care received outside of the USA.	❑ Services by immediate relatives.
❑ Services required as a result of war.	❑ Services under a physician's private contract.

- ❑ Services paid for by a governmental entity that is not Medicare.
- ❑ Services for which the patient has no legal obligation to pay.
- ❑ Home health services furnished under a plan of care, if the agency does not submit the claim.
- ❑ Items and services excluded under the Assisted Suicide Funding Restriction Act of 1997.
- ❑ Items or services furnished in a competitive acquisition area by any entity that does not have a contract with the Department of Health and Human Services (except in a case of urgent need).
- ❑ Physicians' services performed by a physician assistant, midwife, psychologist, or nurse anesthetist, when furnished to an inpatient, unless they are furnished under arrangements by the hospital.
- ❑ Items and services furnished to an individual who is a resident of a skilled nursing facility (a SNF) or of a part of a facility that includes a SNF, unless they are furnished under arrangements by the SNF.
- ❑ Services of an assistant at surgery without prior approval from the peer review organization.
- ❑ Outpatient occupational and physical therapy services furnished incident to a physician's services.

- * **This is only a general summary of exclusions from Medicare benefits. It is not a legal document. The official Medicare program provisions are contained in relevant laws, regulations, and rulings.**

Figure 9–2 Notice of Exclusions from Medicare Benefits (NEMB)

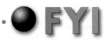
- Too Many Services in a Brief Period of Time—Examples of these denials include more than one office visit in a day, or too many visits for treatment of a minor problem.

- Level of Service Denials—Claims in this category are either denied or downcoded (coded at a lower level) because the services provided were in excess of what was required to adequately diagnose and/or treat the problem. Level of service denials typically occur on claims for office visits. Rather than deny the claim, the payer will downcode the procedure—for example, changing a CPT E/M Level IV code to a Level II code.

A provider who thinks that a procedure will not be covered by Medicare because it will be deemed not reasonable and necessary must notify the patient before the treatment using a standard advance beneficiary notice (ABN) from CMS (see Figure 9.3 on page 156). The ABN form is designed to:

- Identify the service or item that Medicare is unlikely to pay for

- State the reason Medicare is unlikely to pay

- Estimate how much the service or item will cost the beneficiary if Medicare does not pay

ABNs are not required for excluded services; they are only to be used for services that may not be deemed reasonable and necessary by Medicare. As with a NEMB, the purpose of the provider in presenting the patient with the ABN is to help the patient or beneficiary make an informed decision about services he or she might have to pay for out-of-pocket. In addition, if the provider could have been expected to know that a service would not be covered and performed the service without informing the patient, the provider may be liable for the charges.

WHO PAYS FIRST?

Many beneficiaries choose to buy Medigap insurance policies from federally approved private insurance carriers to fill in the gaps in Medicare coverage. Generally, the plan pays the beneficiary's deductibles and coinsurance. Some policies also cover services Medicare does not.

Note that Medicare beneficiaries enrolled in managed care plans usually do not need Medigap insurance. Their plans have the same benefits that Medigap policies offer without an additional premium.

If a beneficiary has Medigap insurance, Medicare is the primary payer. That means Medicare pays first, and then the Medigap carrier determines its obligations. File the claim with Medicare first. Some individuals are eligible for both Medicaid and Medicare (Medi-Medi) benefits. Claims for these patients are first submitted to Medicare. Then they are sent to Medicaid along with the Medicare Remittance Notice. Most Medicare carriers transmit these crossover claims to the state Medicaid payer automatically.

In some situations, Medicare is the secondary payer. Generally, these situations are related to accidents or job-related illnesses or injuries. Medicare is a secondary payer when:

- The patient is covered through an employer's group health plan or the spouse's employer's group health plan.

Patient's Name: _____   Medicare # (HICN): _____

ADVANCE BENEFICIARY NOTICE (ABN)

NOTE: You need to make a choice about receiving these health care items or services.

We expect that Medicare will not pay for the item(s) or service(s) that are described below. Medicare does not pay for all of your health care costs. Medicare only pays for covered items and services when Medicare rules are met. The fact that Medicare may not pay for a particular item or service does not mean that you should not receive it. There may be a good reason your doctor recommended it. Right now, in your case, **Medicare probably will not pay for –**

Items or Services:

Because:

The purpose of this form is to help you make an informed choice about whether or not you want to receive these items or services, knowing that you might have to pay for them yourself. Before you make a decision about your options, you should **read this entire notice carefully.**

- Ask us to explain, if you don't understand why Medicare probably won't pay.
- Ask us how much these items or services will cost you (**Estimated Cost: $_____**), in case you have to pay for them yourself or through other insurance.

PLEASE CHOOSE **ONE** OPTION. CHECK **ONE** BOX. **SIGN & DATE** YOUR CHOICE.

☐ **Option 1. YES.   I want to receive these items or services.**

I understand that Medicare will not decide whether to pay unless I receive these items or services. Please submit my claim to Medicare. I understand that you may bill me for items or services and that I may have to pay the bill while Medicare is making its decision. If Medicare does pay, you will refund to me any payments I made to you that are due to me. If Medicare denies payment, I agree to be personally and fully responsible for payment. That is, I will pay personally, either out of pocket or through any other insurance that I have. I understand I can appeal Medicare's decision.

☐ **Option 2. NO.   I have decided not to receive these items or services.**

I will not receive these items or services. I understand that you will not be able to submit a claim to Medicare and that I will not be able to appeal your opinion that Medicare won't pay.

_____   _____
Date   **Signature of patient or person acting on patient's behalf**

NOTE: Your health information will be kept confidential. Any information that we collect about you on this form will be kept confidential in our offices. If a claim is submitted to Medicare, your health information on this form may be shared with Medicare. Your health information which Medicare sees will be kept confidential by Medicare.

OMB Approval No. 0938-0566   Form No. CMS-R-131-G   (June 2002)

Figure 9–3 Advance Beneficiary Notice (ABN)

Explore the Internet

Visit the Centers for Medicare and Medicaid Services (CMS) Web site for Medicare at http://www.cms.hhs.gov Select the Professionals link (rather than the Consumers link), and then select the Physicians link. Look for information about participating and nonparticipating providers and the Medicare Fee Schedule (MFS). Read the most recent information on that topic. Under the Contacts topic, look up the Medicare Part B carrier(s) for your state.

- The services are for treatment of a work-related illness or injury covered by workers' compensation or federal black lung benefits.
- No-fault insurance or liability insurance covers the services, such as those for illness or injury resulting from an automobile accident.
- A patient with end-stage renal disease is covered by an employer's group health plan. In this case, Medicare is the secondary payer for the first eighteen months.

For Medicare patients in these situations, file first with the other insurance plan and then with Medicare. When completing the Medicare claim, indicate the type of insurance that is primary, using the claim filing indicator code as specified in the HIPAA 837 claim guidelines. The primary remittance advice is sent with the claim to Medicare. Currently, the paper claim (CMS-1500) is used to send secondary claims to Medicare.

Chapter Summary

1. The two parts of Medicare coverage are Part A, which helps pay for inpatient hospital services, care in a skilled nursing facility, home health care, and hospice care; and Part B, which helps pay for physician services, outpatient hospital services, durable medical equipment, and other services and supplies.

2. Medicare fees are developed from the RBRVS system and are listed in the Medicare Fee Schedule. A participating physician accepts the Medicare Fee Schedule as the allowed charge. A nonPAR physician who accepts assignment is paid from the nonparticipating fee schedule, which is 5 percent less than the PAR fee. A nonPAR who does not accept assignment is subject to Medicare's charge limits and may not charge a Medicare patient more than 115 percent of the amount listed in the Medicare nonparticipating fee schedule.

3. An excluded service is one that is never covered by Medicare, while a medically unnecessary service may be covered in the appropriate circumstances. Physicians may use a form such as a Notice of Exclusions from Medicare Benefits to tell patients about excluded services. They are required to use the advance beneficiary notice to inform patients about planned services that Medicare considers medically unnecessary.

4. Medicare is the secondary payer when services are covered by (a) the patient's or spouse's employer's group health plan, (b) workers' compensation or federal black lung benefits, (c) no-fault or liability insurance, or (d) an employer's group health plan for a patient with end-stage renal disease.

Check Your Understanding

Part 1. Write "T" or "F" in the blank to indicate whether you think the statement is true or false.

F **1.** A claim for physician services performed in a hospital setting should be filed under Medicare Part A.

T **2.** A Medicare-participating physician accepts assignment on all Medicare claims.

T **3.** The National Provider Identifier is used for Medicare.

F **4.** Organizations that handle Medicare Part B claims and payments are known as ~~intermediaries~~. *fiscal agents*

T **5.** The Correct Coding Initiative provides guidelines for correct coding of procedures.

T **6.** Medigap plans are secondary payers.

T **7.** Nonparticipating physicians can decide whether to accept assignment on claims on a case-by-case basis.

F **8.** Medicare Advantage is another name for the Medicare Prescription Drug, Improvement, and Modernization Act of 2003 that includes a prescription drug benefit.

F **9.** Participating and nonparticipating physicians are paid using the same fee schedule.

T **10.** Advance beneficiary notices (ABNs) are used exclusively for services that may not be deemed reasonable and necessary by Medicare.

Part 2. Choose the best answer.

B **1.** Medicare is the federal health care plan for:
   a. mothers with preschool-aged children
   (b.) people age sixty-five or older and some disabled people
   c. disadvantaged youth

B **2.** A Medicare beneficiary enrolled in an HMO does not need:
   a. Medicaid
   (b.) a Medigap policy
   c. a MediCal policy

B **3.** HCPCS is a system to identify:
   a. diagnoses
   (b.) procedures
   c. both a and b

B **4.** A Medicare-participating physician may bill a Medicare patient for:
   a. coinsurance
   (b.) excess charges
   c. neither a nor b

a **5.** Medicare is a secondary payer when:
   (a.) services for the treatment of automobile accident injuries are covered by liability insurance
   b. the patient qualifies for Medicaid
   c. the patient subscribes to a Medicare supplemental health insurance plan

6. The payment for a physician's service under Medicare is based on:
   (a.) the amount set by government mandate
   b. an amount based on what the physician usually charges for the service
   c. an amount based on what area physicians usually charge for the service

_____ **7.** If a Medicare beneficiary is covered by an employer's group health plan, Medicare is:
    a. a primary payer
    b. a secondary payer
    c. not in force

_____ **8.** The Medicare fee-for-service plan is known as:
    a. the Original Medicare Plan
    b. the HMO
    c. Medicare Advantage

_____ **9.** The Medicare Modernization Act provides for:
    a. prescription drug coverage
    b. higher coinsurance
    c. more Medigap plans

_____ **10.** Under Medicare Advantage, beneficiaries can choose to enroll in:
    a. Health Savings Accounts
    b. Medicare preferred provider organization plans (PPOs)
    c. both a and b

Part 3. Supply the answers to the following two cases.

A.
Physician Information:
Name: Ralph L. Markarian, MD
NPI: 1234567890
Accepts assignment for Medicare patients

[handwritten: 86 Whatswrong Rd, Providence RI 02906 401-351-4321]

Patient Information Form:
Name: Bonita S. Chavez (Established Patient)
Age: 84
Sex: Female
Birth Date: April 16, 1924
Marital Status: Widowed
Employer: Retired
Medicare ID Number: 221-54-3376C
Additional Insurance Carrier: None

[handwritten: 185 Getthecheckottamy Wy. Providence, RI 02906 401-351-5678]

[handwritten: Medicare, One Weybosset St. Providence, RI 02903]

Patient's Encounter Form:
Date: 5-20-2008
T-98   BP 140/98
CC: Patient visit for diabetes recheck. Off medications for blood pressure and diabetes. Has lost <u>eight</u> pounds since last visit due to change in diet. Discussed diabetes monitoring and lifestyle changes to maintain weight control.
Dx: Type II diabetes. Elevated blood pressure.

List of Fees for Service:
Charges: Level III office visit, $75
No payment collected.
Note: Deductible has been met for 2008.

Supply the following data elements:

Billing Provider _____

Billing Provider's Primary Identifier _____

Subscriber/Patient _____

Subscriber's Primary Identifier _____

Claim Filing Indicator Code _____

Medicare Assignment Code __ (A) Assigned __ C (Not Assigned)

Place of Service Code _____

Diagnosis Codes _____

Total Charge _____

Amount Collected _____

Service Line Information

Date of Service _____

Procedure Code/Charge _____

Diagnosis _____

B.
Physician Information:
Name: William B. Rheingold, MD
NPI: 2345678901
Accepts assignment for Medicare patients

Patient Information Form:
Name: Clair Gibbons (Established Patient)
Sex: Female
Birth Date: July 31, 1935
Marital Status: Single
Employer: Retired
Medicare ID Number: 455-03-7722A
Additional Insurance Carrier: None

Patient's Encounter Form:
Date: October 12, 2008
T-98   BP 120/85
CC: Patient has history of breast cancer; presents with shortness of breath. Ordered chest X-ray in the office, which showed a small pleural effusion on the left. Performed a thoracentesis, drew off fluid; sent for cytology and chemistry analysis.
Dx: Unspecified pleural effusion; personal history of malignant neoplasm of breast.

List of Fees for Service:

Services and Charges:

    Level III office visit, $80

    Thoracentesis, $65

    Radiologic examination, chest, two views, frontal and lateral, $15

    No payment collected.

    Note: Deductible has been met for 2008.

Supply the following data elements:

Billing Provider _____

Billing Provider's Primary Identifier _____

Subscriber/Patient _____

Subscriber's Primary Identifier _____

Claim Filing Indicator Code _____

Medicare Assignment Code __ (A) Assigned __ C (Not Assigned)

Place of Service Code_____

Diagnosis Codes _____

Total Charge _____

Amount Collected _____

Service Line Information

Date of Service _____

Procedure Code/Charge _____

Diagnosis _____

Date of Service _____

Procedure Code/Charge _____

Diagnosis _____

Date of Service _____

Procedure Code/Charge _____

Diagnosis _____

Part 4. The following information is presented on a patient's Medicare MSN. What does the patient owe? _____

BILL SUBMITTED BY: Dr. Anthony B. Starpish
29 Washington Square North
New York, NY 10011

Date	Services and Service Code	Medicare Charges	Approved
2-10-2008	1 Destruction of hemorrhoids (46934-78)	$325.00	$194.78*

(Note: *The approved amount is based on the fee schedule.)

Explanation:

Of the total charges, Medicare approved $194.78   (The provider agreed to accept this amount.)

Your 20 percent   – 38.96

The 80 percent Medicare pays $155.82

You have already met the deductible for 2008.

Part 5. Fill in the blanks in the following payment situations:

Participating Provider

Physician's standard fee	$210.00
Medicare fee	$115.00
Medicare pays 80%	$_____
Patient or supplemental plan pays 20%	$_____
Provider adjustment (write-off)	$_____

Nonparticipating Provider (Accepts Assignment)

Physician's standard fee	$210.00
Medicare nonPAR fee	$109.25
Medicare pays 80%	$_____
Patient/supplemental plan pays 20%	$_____
Provider adjustment (write-off)	$_____

Nonparticipating Provider (Does Not Accept Assignment)

Physician's standard fee	$210.00
Medicare nonPAR fee	$109.25
Limiting charge	$_____
Patient billed	$_____
Medicare pays patient	$_____
Total provider can collect	$_____
Patient out-of-pocket expense	$_____

10 Medicaid

Objectives

After completing this chapter, you will be able to define the key terms and:

1. Identify two ways Medicaid programs vary from state to state.
2. List the primary kinds of Medicaid benefits determined by federal law and give examples of additional benefits that states may authorize.
3. Explain two broad classifications of people who are eligible for Medicaid assistance.
4. Explain four areas a medical insurance specialist should pay special attention to when filing Medicaid claims.

Key Terms

categorically needy
Early and Periodic
    Screening, Diagnosis,
    and Treatment (EPSDT)
Federal Medicaid Assistance
    Percentage (FMAP)

fiscal agent
Medicaid
MediCal
medically indigent
medically needy
payer of last resort

State Children's Health
    Insurance Program (SCHIP)
Temporary Assistance for
    Needy Families (TANF)
third-party liability
Welfare Reform Act

Why This Chapter Is Important to You

The information in this chapter will enable you to:

- Learn who qualifies for Medicaid assistance
- Become familiar with the kinds of medical services covered by Medicaid programs
- Learn important procedures for filing claims for Medicaid patients

What Do You Think?

As an assistance program, Medicaid is federally mandated. However, each state has its own rules and regulations. How can the medical insurance specialist research the state rules that apply? What types of routine or health maintenance services are generally covered by Medicaid?

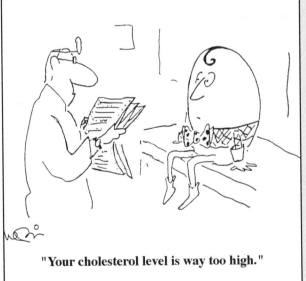

"Your cholesterol level is way too high."

INTRODUCTION TO MEDICAID

M̲ost of the claims that medical insurance specialists file are for benefits due under health insurance plans. However, one government program that pays for health care services is actually an assistance program, not an insurance program.

Medicaid pays for health care services for people with incomes below the national poverty level. Both federal and state governments pay for the program, and in some areas local taxes support it as well. The federal government makes payments to states under the Federal Medicaid Assistance Percentage (FMAP). The amount of the payment is based on the state's average per capita income in relation to the national income average. States with high per capita incomes receive less federal funding than states with low per capita incomes. In each state, Medicaid is administered by a fiscal agent, an organization that processes claims for a government program. The Center for Medicaid and State Operations, a department of the Centers for Medicare and Medicaid Services (CMS), oversees these programs that are administered by the states.

The first Medicaid programs were required by federal law as part of the Social Security Act of 1965. Under the legislation, the federal government determines which kinds of medical services are covered and paid for by the federal portion of the program. States participate in their Medicaid programs in two ways: (1) states may authorize additional kinds of services or make additional groups eligible, and (2) states determine eligibility within federal guidelines. Because of this participation by state governments, Medicaid programs change often and vary widely from state to state. Thus, this chapter gives only general information about Medicaid.

A physician may choose to participate in the Medicaid program or not to accept Medicaid patients. Participating in the Medicaid program means agreeing to accept Medicaid reimbursement for covered services as payment in full. The physician must write off the difference, if any, between fees charged for services and the amount reimbursed. The physician may not bill the patient for the difference. However, the physician may bill the patient for services not covered by Medicaid.

MEDICAID COVERAGE

According to federal guidelines, Medicaid pays for the following types of health care:

- Physician services
- Laboratory and X-ray services
- Inpatient hospital services
- Outpatient hospital services
- Rural health clinic services
- Home health care
- Family planning services
- Federally qualified health-center (FQHC) services
- Skilled care at a public nursing facility

- Prenatal and nurse-midwife services
- Early and Periodic Screening, Diagnosis, and Treatment (EPSDT) services
- Emergency care

Family planning services include counseling, diagnosis, treatment, drugs, and supplies related to planning the number and spacing of children. Early and Periodic Screening, Diagnosis, and Treatment (EPSDT) is a prevention, early-detection, and treatment program for children under the age of twenty-one who are enrolled in Medicaid. Covered services include medical history; physical exam; assessment of development and immunization status; and screening for anemia, lead absorption, tuberculosis, sickle cell trait and disease, and dental, hearing, and vision problems. States must pay for all services identified in an EPSDT exam, whether or not they pay for the service for other eligible individuals.

The State Children's Health Insurance Program (SCHIP), part of the Balanced Budget Act of 1997, requires states to develop and implement plans for health insurance coverage for uninsured children. The more than 5 million children served by SCHIP come from low-income families, but the incomes are not low enough to qualify for Medicaid. The program is funded jointly by the federal government and the states. It provides coverage for many preventive services and covers children up to age nineteen.

The Ticket to Work and Work Incentives Improvement Act of 1999 (TWWIIA) expands the availability of health care services for workers with disabilities. Previously, persons with disabilities often had to choose between health care and work. TWWIIA gives states the option of allowing individuals with disabilities to purchase Medicaid coverage that is necessary to enable them to maintain employment.

The state portion of a Medicaid program often includes a number of additional services under its federally funded Medicaid program. Some examples of extra assistance enacted by individual states include:

- Clinic services
- Emergency room care
- Ambulance services
- Chiropractic services
- Mental-health services
- Certain cosmetic procedures
- Allergy services
- Dermatology services
- Dental care
- Home and community-based care to certain persons with chronic impairments.
- Podiatry services
- Eyeglasses and eye refractions
- Prescription drugs
- Prosthetic devices
- Private-duty nursing
- Other diagnostic, screening, preventive, and rehabilitative services

In recent years, however, because of large state budget deficits, state laws have cut back on some of these benefits—for example, prescription drug benefits and hearing, vision, and dental benefits for adults. Many states have also had to restrict eligibility for Medicaid and to reduce Medicaid payments to doctors, hospitals, nursing homes, or other providers.

In each state, the Medicaid and/or social services agency can provide a list of services and any limits or preauthorization requirements for those services. Any additional services, such as those just listed, are paid entirely from state funds.

Professional Focus

Medicaid Fraud and Abuse

The Medicaid Alliance for Program Safeguards is committed to fighting fraud and abuse, which divert dollars that should be spent to safeguard the health and welfare of Medicaid clients. Although states are primarily responsible for policing fraud in the Medicaid program, CMS provides technical assistance, guidance, and oversight in these efforts. Fraud schemes often cross state lines, and CMS strives to improve information sharing among the Medicaid programs and other stakeholders.

Medicaid fraud can take many forms. Here are some of the more common schemes:

- Billing for "phantom patients" who did not really receive services.
- Billing for medical services or goods that were not provided.
- Billing for old items as if they were new.
- Billing for more hours than there are in a day.
- Billing for tests that the patient did not need.
- Paying a kickback in exchange for a referral for medical services or goods.
- Charging Medicaid for personal expenses not related to caring for a Medicaid client.
- Overcharging for health care services or goods that were provided.
- Concealing ownership in a related company.
- Using false credentials.
- Double-billing for health care services or goods that were provided.

MEDICAID ELIGIBILITY

Generally, Medicaid recipients are people with low incomes who have children or are over the age of sixty-five, are blind, or have permanent disabilities. Within federal guidelines, states determine income levels and other qualifications for eligibility.

One group of Medicaid recipients is known as categorically needy. Their needs are addressed under the Personal Responsibility and Work Opportunity Reconciliation Act of 1996 (P.L. 104-193), commonly known as the Welfare Reform Act, which created Temporary Assistance for Needy Families (TANF). Eligibility for TANF is determined at the county level. These programs help with living, as opposed to medical, expenses.

Some states extend Medicaid eligibility to include another group of people classified as medically needy or medically indigent. These individuals earn enough money to pay for basic living expenses, but they cannot afford high medical bills. In some cases, Medicaid recipients in the medically needy classification must pay deductibles before they receive benefits. Some Medicaid recipients in this category must pay coinsurance for medical services. States choose their own names for these programs. For example, California calls this program MediCal.

Once Medicaid eligibility is determined, the recipient gets an identification card or coupon explaining effective dates and additional information such as a coinsurance requirement, if any. Different states authorize coverage for different lengths of time. Some states issue cards twice a month, some once a month, and others every two months or every six months. Most states, however, are moving to electronic verification of eligibility under the Electronic Medicaid Eligibility Verification System (EMEVS). Patients' eligibility should be checked each time they make an appointment and before they see the physician. Many states provide both online and telephone verification systems.

FILING MEDICAID CLAIMS

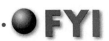

Medicaid claims are filed in the patient's home state. Because Medicaid is covered by HIPAA, Medicaid claims are usually submitted using the HIPAA 837 claim (see Chapter 6). In some situations, however, a paper claim using the CMS-1500 format may be used, or a state-specific form may be requested. HCPCS codes are used for the procedures. In each state, the fiscal agent provides the rules for submitting claims.

Medicaid managed care claims are filed differently than other Medicaid claims. Claims are sent to the managed care organization instead of to the state Medicaid department. Participating providers agree to the guidelines of the managed care organization, provided that they are in compliance with federal requirements.

Sometimes a physician in one state treats a patient who lives in another state, either because the patient is traveling or because the patient lives near a state boundary and has easier access to physicians in a neighboring state. Since Medicaid is administered on a state-by-state basis, the Medicaid claim must be filed in the patient's home state. Nevertheless, most Medicaid programs have state-to-state agreements to cover each other's Medicaid patients. The fiscal agent in the patient's home state may be contacted to get forms and claim processing information.

When filing Medicaid claims for any state, the medical insurance specialist should pay special attention to:

- Eligibility—Medicaid eligibility varies from month to month if the recipient's income fluctuates. Comply with the state's requirements for verifying eligibility. Check the patient's Medicaid identification card or coupon, and photocopy the front and back on each visit. Date the photocopy. Some states require this photocopy to be attached to the submitted claim form. An example of a Medicaid card is shown in Figure 10-1 on page 170.

- Preauthorization—Most states require preauthorization for specified services. Check with the state's fiscal agent to find out how to get preauthorization by telephone and whether a written confirmation form must also be filed. If the state requires

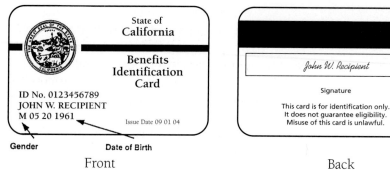

Figure 10-1 Sample Medicaid Card

preauthorization, charges for services that did not get prior approval will not be paid. In emergencies, such as emergency room situations, authorization may be obtained after the treatment.

- Filing Deadline—The time line for filing a Medicaid claim ranges from two months to one year from the date of service. Find out the state's requirements, and file claims promptly.
- Third-Party Liability—Third-party liability is the obligation of a government program or insurance plan to pay all or part of a patient's medical costs. Before filing a claim with Medicaid, it is important to determine whether the patient has other insurance coverage.

If a patient who is eligible for Medicaid has additional health care coverage through an insurance plan or another government program such as Medicare, the patient's Medicaid eligibility does not relieve the other program or plan of its responsibility. In fact, the other program or insurance carrier is the primary carrier in these cases. Medicaid is the secondary carrier. File the claim first with the primary carrier, and file for Medicaid benefits last. Because of this sequence, Medicaid is referred to as the payer of last resort.

Chapter Summary

1. Medicaid programs differ among states in the services covered and the way eligibility is determined.

2. The federal government requires all states, as participants in the Medicaid program, to provide at least the following services to the categorically needy: (a) physician services; (b) laboratory and X-ray services; (c) inpatient hospital services; (d) outpatient hospital services; (e) rural health clinic services; (f) home health care; (g) family planning services; (h) federally qualified health-center (FQHC) services; (i) skilled care at a public nursing facility; (j) prenatal and nurse-midwife services; (k) Early and Periodic Screening, Diagnosis, and Treatment (EPSDT) services, and (l) emergency care. A state may fund additional services for the categorically needy and may choose to pay for services to the medically needy. Some states may also have medical general assistance programs that provide services to individuals not eligible for the federal Medicaid program.

3. Two broad classifications of people who are eligible for Medicaid are the categorically needy and medically needy or medically indigent.

4. The four areas a medical insurance specialist should pay particular attention to when filing Medicaid claims are eligibility, preauthorization, filing deadline, and third-party liability.

Check Your Understanding

Part 1. Fill in the answer to each question. Some answers have more than one word.

1. A government program that helps pay living expenses for low-income families and children is known as _____ _____ _____ _____ _____.

2. People who qualify for federal government programs for living expenses are classified as _____ needy.

3. The longest time limit for filing Medicaid claims is one _____ from the date of service.

4. The obligation of a government program or insurance plan to pay all or part of a patient's medical costs is _____ liability.

5. EPSDT services are for children _____ than the age of twenty-one.

6. One of the services authorized for payment with EPSDT funds is a physical _____.

7. In California the Medicaid program is called _____.

8. Medicaid is an assistance program for people with a _____ who are aged, blind, disabled, or pregnant, and for members of their families.

9. EPSDT stands for _____ Screening, Diagnosis, and Treatment.

10. Some Medicaid recipients must pay deductibles and _____.

11. Medicaid programs must pay for both outpatient and _____ hospital care for the categorically needy.

12. Within federal guidelines, states determine who is _____ for Medicaid.

13. The federal government revised the rules covering Medicaid eligibility in the _____ Reform Act.

14. SCHIP stands for the _____ Health Insurance Program.

15. FMAP is a _____ program that determines how Medicaid payments are made to the states.

16. If the patient is eligible for Medicaid but has additional health coverage, the other program is the _____ payer.

17. Medicaid is called the _____ of last resort.

18. The _____ coding system is used to report procedures on Medicaid claims.

19. Because Medicaid is under HIPAA, Medicaid claims are usually submitted using the _____ claim.

20. The _____ program covers recipients under age twenty-one who need screening and diagnostic services.

Part 2. Supply the answers to the following two cases.

A.
Physician Information:
Name: Selena R. Rodez, MD
NPI: 8901234567
Medicaid PIN: HC29004

Patient Information Form:
Name: Grace B. Chin (New Patient)
Age: 43
Sex: Female
Birth Date: November 7, 1963
Social Security Number: 056-99-0034
Medicaid Eligibility: June 1-30, 2008 (*Note:* Copayment of $10 per office visit required.)
Medicaid Number: 056990034
Insurance Carrier: None

Patient's Encounter Form:
Date: 6-20-2008
T-98   BP 135/80
CC: Patient has cut in the white part of her eye, cause unknown. No visual problems. Reports some pain.
Dx: Eyeball abrasion, left eye.
Rx: Ophthalmic solution, 2 drops to right eye × 10 days.

List of Fees for Service:
Charges: Office visit, Level I, $35
Copayment collected

Supply the following data elements:

Billing Provider _____

Billing Provider's Primary Identifier _____

Billing Provider's Secondary Identifier _____

Subscriber/Patient _____

Subscriber's Primary Identifier _____

Claim Filing Indicator Code _____

Place of Service Code _____

Diagnosis Codes _____

Total Charge _____

Amount Collected _____

Service Line Information

Date of Service _____

Procedure Code/Charge _____

Diagnosis _____

B.
Physician Information:
Name: Gloria A. Poyner, MD
NPI: 9012345678
Medicaid PIN: DC55289

Patient Information Form:
Name: George Eustis Kador (New Patient)
Sex: Male
Birth Date: November 27, 1948
Social Security Number: 033-45-7034
Medicaid Eligibility: July 1-31, 2008 (Note: Copayment of $7.50 per office visit required.)
Medicaid Number: 046971134
Insurance Carrier: None

Patient's Encounter Form:
Date: 7-7-2008
T-98 BP 135/80
CC: Patient presents with complaint of recent onset of palpitations. Reviewed social and medical history and records. Performed detailed system review and prescribed a twenty-four-hour electrocardiographic monitoring (a continuous original ECG waveform), supplying the monitor with hookup and recording; scanning analysis with report; reviewed and interpreted the analysis and report.
Dx: Palpitations

Date: 7-8-2008
Follow-up Office Visit: Diagnosed ectopic auricular beats. Discussed therapy with patient in this follow-up visit.
Dx: Supraventricular premature beats

List of Fees for Services
7-7-2008
Services and Charges: Office visit, comprehensive history, comprehensive examination, moderately complex medical decision making, $65
ECG monitoring for twenty-four hours—recording, analysis/report, physician analysis and interpretation, $125
Copayment collected

7-8-2008
Services and Charges: Office visit, expanded history and examination, fifteen minutes with patient, $45
Copayment collected

Supply the following data elements:

Billing Provider _____

Billing Provider's Primary Identifier _____

Billing Provider's Secondary Identifier _____

Subscriber/Patient _____

Subscriber's Primary Identifier _____

Claim Filing Indicator Code _____

Place of Service Code _____

Diagnosis Codes _____

Total Charge _____

Amount Collected _____

Service Line Information

Date of Service _____

Procedure Code/Charge _____

Diagnosis _____

Date of Service _____

Procedure Code/Charge _____

Diagnosis _____

Date of Service _____

Procedure Code/Charge _____

Diagnosis _____

11 TRICARE and CHAMPVA

Objectives

After completing this chapter, you will be able to define the key terms and:

1. Explain who is eligible for TRICARE and CHAMPVA and how to verify eligibility.
2. Discuss the three programs offered to TRICARE beneficiaries.
3. Describe the use of a nonavailability statement in the TRICARE program.
4. Explain where to file claims first when TRICARE and CHAMPVA beneficiaries are also covered by other insurance programs.
5. Identify filing deadlines and time limits for responses to requests for additional information.

Key Terms

catastrophic cap
CHAMPVA
CHAMPVA for Life
cost-share
Defense Enrollment Eligibility
  Reporting System (DEERS)

military treatment facility
  (MTF)
nonavailability statement
  (NAS)
Primary Care Manager
  (PCM)

sponsor
TRICARE
TRICARE Extra
TRICARE for Life
TRICARE Prime
TRICARE Standard

176

Why This Chapter Is Important to You

The information in this chapter will enable you to:
- Know who qualifies for military health care programs
- Know where to send beneficiaries for answers to insurance coverage and claim questions
- File TRICARE and CHAMPVA claims

What Do You Think?

TRICARE and CHAMPVA are government medical insurance plans primarily for families of members of the U.S. uniformed services. Special regulations apply to situations in which beneficiaries seek medical services outside of military treatment facilities. What are the best ways to find out about the rules and regulations pertaining to these patients?

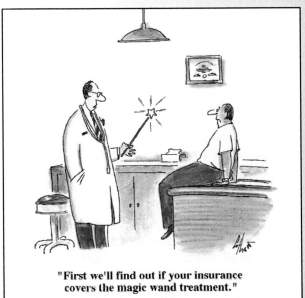

"First we'll find out if your insurance covers the magic wand treatment."

TRICARE is the Department of Defense's health insurance plan for military personnel and their families. TRICARE offers three different health care plans to its beneficiaries in the Army, Navy, Air Force, Marine Corps, Coast Guard, Public Health Service, and National Oceanic and Atmospheric Administration. TRICARE replaced the program known as CHAMPUS (Civilian Health and Medical Program of the Uniformed Services).

TRICARE benefits spouses and children of active-duty service members, who are called sponsors. The health care for the service members themselves is automatically provided or paid for by their branch of service. TRICARE also serves military retirees and their families, some former spouses, and survivors of deceased military members.

A TRICARE beneficiary must be listed in the Department of Defense's Defense Enrollment Eligibility Reporting System (DEERS). DEERS is a worldwide database of people covered by TRICARE. DEERS helps the Department of Defense track the use of medical services to better plan for beneficiaries' needs. It also helps eliminate fraudulent use of military benefits.

TRICARE Standard

TRICARE Standard is a fee-for-service program. The program covers medical services provided by a civilian physician when the individual cannot receive treatment from a military treatment facility (MTF). Military families may receive services at an MTF, but the services offered vary by facility, and first priority is given to active-duty service members. When service is not available, the individual seeks treatment from a civilian provider, and TRICARE Standard benefits go into effect.

TRICARE Standard pays for most of the costs of medically necessary services, which are primarily provided in military hospitals. Individuals must first seek care at a military treatment facility. If an individual lives within a certain proximity to a military hospital, generally within a forty-mile radius, a nonavailability statement (NAS) must be filed by the local military hospital before the patient can be treated at a civilian hospital for inpatient nonemergency care. The NAS is an electronic document stating that the service the patient requires is not available at the nearby military treatment facility. The form is electronically transmitted to the DEERS database. If it is not filed, TRICARE will not pay the hospital claim. If the patient has other insurance that is primary to TRICARE, an NAS is not required. In addition, emergency services do not require a nonavailability statement.

Under TRICARE Standard, medical expenses are shared between TRICARE and the beneficiary. The TRICARE program uses the term cost-share for the patient's responsibility for coinsurance. Patient cost-share payments are subject to an annual catastrophic cap, a limit on the total medical expenses that the patient must pay in one year. Once this cap has been met, TRICARE pays 100 percent of additional charges for that coverage year.

> **✓ Compliance Tip**
>
> TRICARE Standard does not require outpatient nonavailability statements except in the case of outpatient prenatal and postpartum maternity care. Most high-cost procedures do require preauthorization, however. Medical information specialists should contact their TRICARE contractor for specific information.

TRICARE Prime

TRICARE Prime is a managed care plan similar to an HMO. After enrolling in the plan, each individual is assigned a Primary Care Manager (PCM) who coordinates and manages that patient's medical care. The PCM may be a single military or civilian provider, or a group of providers. In addition to most of the benefits offered by TRICARE Standard, the program offers preventive care, including routine physical examinations. Active-duty service members are automatically enrolled in TRICARE Prime. TRICARE Prime enrollees receive the majority of their health care services from military treatment facilities, and they receive priority at these facilities.

An individual must pay an annual enrollment fee to join the TRICARE Prime program. Under TRICARE Prime, there is no deductible, and no payment is required for outpatient treatment at a military facility. For active-duty family members, no payment is required for visits to civilian network providers, but for other beneficiaries, different copayments apply depending on the type of visit. For example, for retirees and their family members, outpatient visits with a civilian provider require a $12 copayment.

TRICARE Extra

TRICARE Extra is an alternative managed care plan for individuals who want to receive services primarily from civilian facilities and physicians rather than military facilities. Since it is a managed care plan, individuals must receive health care services from a select network of health care professionals. They may also seek treatment at a military facility, but active-duty personnel and other TRICARE Prime enrollees receive priority at those facilities, so care may not always be available. TRICARE Extra is more expensive than TRICARE Prime, but less costly than TRICARE Standard. There is no enrollment fee, but there is an annual deductible.

Professional Focus

TRICARE and the HIPPA Privacy Rule

The Military Health System (MHS) and the TRICARE health plan are required to comply with the HIPAA privacy policies and procedures for the use and disclosure of PHI. The MHS's Notice of Privacy Practices, which describes how a patient's medical information may be used and disclosed and how a patient can access the information, is posted at the TRICARE Web site at http://www.tricare.osd.mil.hipaa/

The HIPAA Electronic Health Care Transaction and Code Sets requirements, as well as the Security Rule, must also be followed.

CHAMPVA

CHAMPVA is the Civilian Health and Medical Program of the Veterans Administration, which is now known as the Department of Veterans Affairs. This government program helps pay health care costs for families of veterans who are totally and permanently disabled because of service-related injuries. It also covers the surviving spouse and children of a veteran who died from a service-related disability. Some surviving spouses of a service member who died on active duty may be eligible for CHAMPVA.

The Veterans Health Care Eligibility Reform Act of 1996 requires veterans with a 100 percent disability to be enrolled in the program to receive benefits. Prior to this legislation, enrollment was not required. The Department of Veterans Affairs determines eligibility. CHAMPVA enrollees do not need to obtain nonavailability statements, as they are not eligible to receive service in a military treatment facility. A VA hospital is not considered a military treatment facility.

BENEFICIARY IDENTIFICATION

People who qualify for TRICARE or CHAMPVA are called beneficiaries. Beneficiaries get identification cards that contain information needed for claim forms (see Figure 11-1). When a patient qualifies for one of these programs, the medical insurance specialist checks the effective and expiration dates to be sure that the card authorizes civilian medical care. Then a photocopy of the front and back of the identification card is filed in the patient's medical record. If a patient is a child under the age of ten, the parent's card is checked; beneficiaries under the age of ten usually do not get identification cards.

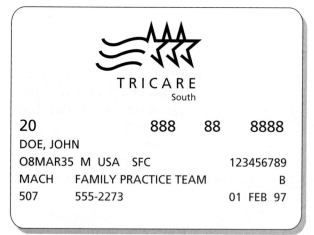
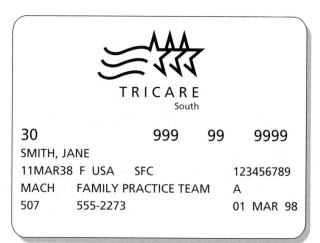

Figure 11-1 Sample Military Health Insurance Identification Card

Although the claim processor needs eligibility information from the DEERS system, there are times when a beneficiary is not listed. For example, even though military sponsors must enroll their families in DEERS, sometimes the sponsors do not keep up with changes in family status or location. Also, new service members may not have had time to enroll their families.

The medical insurance specialist should ask all TRICARE and CHAMPVA patients whether they are enrolled in DEERS. Patients can check their status through the nearest personnel office of any branch of service or through the toll-free number of the DEERS center.

BILLING BENEFICIARIES

HIPAA Tip

Sponsors may telephone DEERS to verify eligibility; providers may not contact DEERS directly because the information is protected by the HIPAA Privacy Rule.

TRICARE pays only for services rendered by authorized providers. Authorized providers are certified by TRICARE regional contractors as having met specific requirements, and each is assigned a PIN. Providers then must decide whether to participate.

Participating physicians must accept assignment—that is, patients may not be billed for more than the allowed charges for covered services. Participating physicians must also file the claims for the patients. Payments on assigned claims are made directly to physicians by the regional TRICARE contractor.

A physician who does not participate has the option to accept assignment on a case-by-case basis. When the physician does not accept assignment, the TRICARE beneficiary is billed for the total actual charge. In this case, the beneficiary is responsible for filing the claim. The beneficiary is also responsible for paying any difference between the allowed amount and the charge. Thus, reimbursement for a nonassigned claim goes to the beneficiary.

Generally, CHAMPVA does not contract with providers. Beneficiaries may receive care from the provider of their choosing as long as that provider is properly licensed to perform the services being delivered. Providers who treat CHAMPVA patients are prohibited from charging more than the CHAMPVA allowable amounts. Providers agree to accept the CHAMPVA payment and the patient's cost-share payment as payment in full for services.

Filing for TRICARE Benefits

Participating providers file claims on behalf of patients. Claims are filed with the contractor for their region. Claims are submitted to the regional contractor based on the patient's home address, not the location of the facility providing the service. Contact information for regional contractors is available on the TRICARE Web site. In 2003, in an effort to simplify the administration of the TRICARE program, the Department of Defense made plans to collapse its eleven administration regions into three (see Figure 11-2). The new regions, phased in during 2004, are referred to as TRICARE North, TRICARE

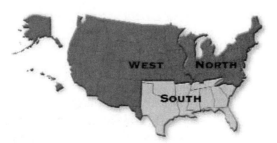

Figure 11-2 TRICARE Regions Map

South, and TRICARE West. Each region is represented by one of three TRICARE contractors selected to replace the previous seven contractors. The exact perimeters of each region may change, so it is important to verify a region through the TRICARE Web site before submitting claims.

Individuals file their own claims when services are received from a non-participating provider, using DD Form 2642, Patient's Request for Medical Payment. A copy of the itemized bill from the provider must be attached to the form. This bill must include the following information:

- Physician's name
- Physician's address
- Physician identification number
- Beneficiary/patient's name
- Date of service
- Procedure code(s) or clear description of service(s)
- Number of services provided
- Diagnosis
- Place of service
- Charge for each service
- Sponsor's Social Security number

Filing for CHAMPVA Benefits

Most CHAMPVA claims are filed by the provider and submitted to the centralized CHAMPVA claims processing center in Denver, Colorado. The information required on a claim is the same as the information required for TRICARE. As with TRICARE, the CHAMPVA program is covered by HIPAA regulations.

When beneficiaries are filing their own claims, the CHAMPVA Claim Form (VA Form 10-7959A) must be used. The claim must always be accompanied by an itemized bill from the provider.

PRIMARY OR SECONDARY PAYER?

TRICARE and CHAMPVA do not duplicate benefits from another insurance program or health plan. The medical insurance specialist must know where to file claims when a beneficiary has additional coverage from Medicaid, supplemental insurance, another health plan, workers' compensation, or Medicare.

If a beneficiary qualifies for Medicaid or has coverage from a supplemental insurance policy (similar to Medigap policies discussed in Chapter 9), TRICARE or CHAMPVA is the primary payer. File with TRICARE or CHAMPVA first. On the other hand, TRICARE and CHAMPVA are secondary payers when the patient has coverage from another primary health plan. For example, a CHAMPVA member (but not a TRICARE member) may be enrolled in Medicare Parts A and B. In this case, Medicare receives the claim first. Then a copy of the MRN or other remittance advice is attached to the CHAMPVA claim.

TRICARE and CHAMPVA do not pay for illnesses or injuries covered by workers' compensation unless compensation benefits have been exhausted. File a workers' compensation claim first (see Chapter 12).

TRICARE and Medicare

The TRICARE for Life plan offers health care at a military treatment facility to individuals age sixty-five and over who are eligible for both Medicare and TRICARE. TRICARE for Life acts as a secondary payer to Medicare; Medicare pays first, and the remaining out-of-pocket expenses are paid by TRICARE. Claims are filed automatically.

Benefits are similar to those of a Medicare HMO, with an emphasis on preventive and wellness services. Prescription drug benefits are also included. All enrollees in TRICARE for Life must be enrolled in Medicare Parts A and B and must have Part B premiums deducted from their Social Security checks. (Individuals already enrolled in a Medicare HMO may not participate in TRICARE for Life.) Other than Medicare costs, TRICARE for Life beneficiaries pay no enrollment fees and no cost-share fees for inpatient or outpatient care at a military facility. Treatment at a civilian network facility requires a copay.

CHAMPVA and Medicare

CHAMPVA for Life extends CHAMPVA benefits to spouses or dependents who are age sixty-five and over. Similar to TRICARE for Life, CHAMPVA for Life benefits are payable after payment by Medicare or other third-party payers. Eligible beneficiaries must be sixty-five or older and enrolled in Medicare Parts A and B. For services not covered by Medicare, such as outpatient prescription medications, CHAMPVA acts as the primary payer.

Filing Forms on Time

TRICARE and CHAMPVA claims must be filed within one year from the date services were provided. For example, a claim for services performed on December 31, 2007, must be filed by December 31, 2008. Of course, medical insurance claims are usually filed more promptly. If an unusual situation occurs, the medical insurance specialist should contact the fiscal intermediary for the area to be sure of complying with this deadline. If additional information is requested, the claim must be resubmitted either within ninety days of the notice or by the regular filing deadline, whichever is later.

Explore the Internet

Visit the official government Web site for TRICARE at http://www.tricare.osd.mil Locate the TRICARE Beneficiaries information section. From the list of options, select TRICARE Resources and then TRICARE Handbook. From the list of Browse subjects, read about the topic Medicare and TRICARE in the TRICARE Handbook. Then return to the TRICARE Beneficiaries information section, and study eligibility requirements and covered services.

Chapter Summary

1. TRICARE serves active duty personnel, their spouses and children, military retirees and their families, some former spouses, and survivors of deceased military members. CHAMPVA covers families of veterans who have service-related 100 percent disabilities and the surviving spouses and children of veterans who have died from service-related injuries. A medical insurance specialist determines eligibility by checking the beneficiary's identification card and verifying that the beneficiary is enrolled in the Defense Enrollment Eligibility Reporting System (DEERS).

2. TRICARE Standard is a fee-for-service plan in which medical expenses are shared between TRICARE and the beneficiary. Most enrollees pay an annual deductible and a cost-share percentage. TRICARE Prime is a managed care plan. After enrolling in the plan, each individual is assigned a Primary Care Manager (PCM) who coordinates and manages that patient's medical care. TRICARE Extra is also a managed care plan, but instead of services being provided primarily from military facilities, civilian facilities and physicians provide the majority of care.

3. When an individual lives within a certain distance from a military hospital, a nonavailability statement (NAS) must be filed by the local military hospital before the patient enters the civilian hospital for non-emergency inpatient care.

4. File first with TRICARE or CHAMPVA when a beneficiary is also covered by Medicaid or supplemental insurance. File a secondary claim with TRICARE or CHAMPVA when the beneficiary has another health plan or when workers' compensation benefits are exhausted.

5. The filing deadline for TRICARE and CHAMPVA claims is one year from the date of service. Requested additional information must be resubmitted within ninety days of the claim processor's request or by the original filing deadline, whichever is later.

Check Your Understanding

Part 1. Write short answers to the following questions.

1. What is the difference between TRICARE and CHAMPVA?

2. What are two benefits of DEERS?

3. What are the three main programs of TRICARE?

4. The physician who employs you is a participating physician with TRICARE. Elaine Dempsey is a new patient in the medical office. She is covered by Blue Cross and Blue Shield through her employer. However, her husband is in the Navy, stationed at Mystic, Connecticut. How should Elaine's claim be filed?

Part 2. **In the space provided, write the word or phrase that best completes each sentence.**

1. The maximum amount a TRICARE beneficiary must pay for deductible and cost-share each year is called the _____.

2. The worldwide database of TRICARE beneficiaries is called _____ .

3. TRICARE Standard is a _____ plan.

4. The name for the uniformed service member in a family qualified for TRICARE or CHAMPVA is _____.

5. The two TRICARE managed care plans are _____ and _____.

6. Coinsurance for a TRICARE or CHAMPVA beneficiary is called the _____.

7. The health care program for active-duty service members, spouses and children of active-duty service members, military retirees and their families, some former spouses, and survivors of deceased military members is called _____.

8. The filing deadline for TRICARE and CHAMPVA claims is _____.

9. TRICARE Prime requires a _____ to be assigned to patients.

10. The DEERS system is administered by _____.

Part 3. **Supply the answers to the following two cases.**

A.
Physician Information:
Name: Asha Gupta, MD
NPI: 5432109876
TRICARE PAR
CHAMPUS (TRICARE) ID: HL59004

Patient Information Form:
Name: Mary Amy Piotrowska (Established Patient)
Sex: Female
Birth Date: 7-5-83
Marital Status: Married
Social Security Number: 031-10-7944

Insurance Information:
Primary Insurance Carrier: TRICARE Standard
Insurance ID Number: 565-97-9087
Insurance Group Number: 565-97-9087 (N4441514)
Secondary Carrier: None
ID Card: EFF 10-10-2007 EXP 10-10-2008

Policyholder Information:
Primary Policyholder: Alfred R. Piotrowska
Employer: U.S. Navy
Address: USS Newport, Box 39
         Sarasota, Florida 33580
Active Duty, Captain
Social Security Number: 565-97-9087
Sex: Male
Birth Date: 6-10-81

Patient's Encounter Form:

Date: 6-25-2008

T-99.7   BP 130/90

CC: Patient reports stuffy nose, sore throat, and low-grade fever.

Dx: Sinusitis.

List of Fees for Service:

Charges: Office visit, Level II (total time, ten minutes), $45

No payment collected.

Supply the following data elements:

Billing Provider _____

Billing Provider's Primary Identifier _____

Billing Provider's Secondary Identifier _____

Subscriber _____

Patient _____

Subscriber's Primary Identifier _____

Relationship _____

Claim Filing Indicator Code _____

Payer Name/ID _____

Place of Service Code _____

Diagnosis Codes _____

Total Charge _____

Amount Collected _____

Service Line Information

Date of Service _____

Procedure Code/Charge _____

Diagnosis _____

B.

Physician Information:
Name: Rory Mancinni, MD
NPI: 3210987654
TRICARE PAR
CHAMPUS (TRICARE) ID: LR33205

Patient Information:
Name: Mary Beth Carteret (Established Patient)
Sex: Female
Birth Date: 12-3-2007
Marital Status: Single
Social Security Number: 066-15-6664

Insurance Information:
Primary Insurance Carrier: TRICARE Prime
Insurance ID Number: 230-77-9987
Insurance Group Number: 230-77-9987 (AF2233)
Secondary Carrier: None
ID Card: EFF 11-10-2007 EXP 11-10-2008

Policyholder Information:
Primary Policyholder: Alice Carteret
Employer: U.S. Air Force
Address: Culver Air Force Base
             Carson, North Carolina 27560
Active Duty, Major
Social Security Number: 230-77-9987
Sex: Female
Birth Date: 4-17-76

Patient's Encounter Form:
Date: 6-25-2008
T-99.7   BP 130/90
CC: Ms. Carteret presents her child for a routine health check and a scheduled DPT + polio immunization.
Dx: Routine infant health check. Need for prophylactic vaccination with diphtheria-tetanus-pertussis with poliomyelitis vaccine.

List of Fees for Services:
Services and Charges: Office visit (periodic preventive medicine reevaluation), $45
        DPT, immunization, active, $7
        Poliomyelitis vaccine, immunization, active, $5
No payment collected

Supply the following data elements:

Billing Provider _____

Billing Provider's Primary Identifier _____

Billing Provider's Secondary Identifier _____

Subscriber _____

Patient _____

Subscriber's Primary Identifier _____

Relationship _____

Claim Filing Indicator Code _____

Payer Name/ID _____

Place of Service Code _____

Diagnosis Codes _____

Total Charge _____

Amount Collected _____

Service Line Information

Date of Service _____

Procedure Code/Charge _____

Diagnosis _____

Date of Service _____

Procedure Code/Charge _____

Diagnosis _____

Date of Service _____

Procedure Code/Charge _____

Diagnosis _____

12 Workers' Compensation

Objectives

After completing this chapter, you will be able to define the key terms and:

1. Discuss what workers' compensation insurance covers, and tell which federal and state agencies administer the programs.
2. List the five types of compensation that employees may receive for work-related illnesses and injuries.
3. List five questions to ask the state compensation board about workers' compensation regulations.
4. Explain why medical information that pertains to a workers' compensation case should be separated from the patient's chart for diseases and disorders that are not work-related.

Key Terms

Federal Employees'
 Compensation Act (FECA)
final report
first report of injury or illness
nontraumatic injury
occupational disease or
 illness

Office of Workers'
 Compensation Programs
 (OWCP)
progress report
state compensation board or
 commission

supplemental report
traumatic injury
workers' compensation
 insurance

Why This Chapter Is Important to You

The information in this chapter will enable you to:

- Know what to do if a patient with a work-related injury or illness comes to your medical office
- Know where to call for more information about state or federal workers' compensation insurance
- Understand the importance of filing claim forms and other medical information for patients with work-related injuries or illnesses

What Do You Think?

Workers' compensation coverage provides important medical insurance benefits to people who experience work-related injuries or illnesses. Unfortunately, many instances of abuse of workers' compensation have been uncovered. In a significant number of these situations, workers' claims for temporary or permanent disability have been found untruthful in court cases. Do medical office staff have a responsibility to question or report information they suspect is fraudulent?

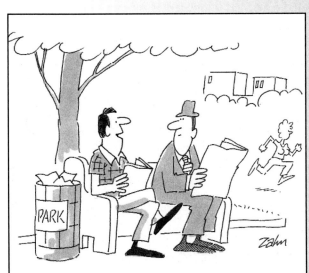

"I'm getting worker's compensation from the Street Department. The shovel I was leaning on broke."

WHEN EMPLOYEES ARE HURT AT WORK

When someone is injured accidentally in the course of performing work or a work-related duty or becomes ill as a result of the employment environment, the cost of medical care for the injury or illness is covered by federal or state plans known as workers' compensation insurance. These plans also provide benefits for lost wages and permanent disabilities.

Workers' compensation covers two kinds of situation that require medical care. A traumatic injury is caused by a specific event or series of events within a single workday or shift. An example is a broken leg caused by a fall from a catwalk in a warehouse. Occupational disease or illness (also known as nontraumatic injury) is caused by the work environment over a longer period of time. An example of an occupational disease is a lung condition caused by repeated exposure to fumes in the workplace.

Compensation for work-related illnesses and injuries may be one of five types:

- Medical treatment
- Lost wages (temporary disability)
- Permanent disability payments (either partial or full disability)
- Compensation for dependents of employees who are fatally injured
- Vocational rehabilitation

FEDERAL PROGRAMS, FORMS, AND PROCEDURES

Work-related illnesses or injuries suffered by civilian employees of federal agencies, including volunteers in the Peace Corps and VISTA, are covered under the Federal Employees' Compensation Act (FECA). Other federal workers' compensation laws include the Federal Coal Mine Health and Safety Act (which includes the Black Lung Benefits Act), the Longshore and Harbor Workers' Compensation Act, and the Energy Employees Occupational Illness Compensation Program Act. All of these plans are administered by the Office of Workers' Compensation Programs (OWCP), except for the Longshore and Harbor Workers' Compensation Act, which is administered by the Division of Longshore and Harbor Workers. Both the OWCP and the Division of Longshore and Harbor Workers are part of the U.S. Department of Labor.

Injured federal employees can choose a physician from among those who are authorized by the OWCP. When such a patient requests treatment, the medical insurance specialist should verify that the selected physician is authorized to administer medical care under the patient's workers' compensation coverage. If the patient later wants to change physicians, the OWCP must approve the change. If a patient seeks care from an unauthorized physician, the medical insurance specialist should remind the patient that he or she may be responsible for the cost of that treatment.

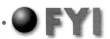

The Occupational Safety and Health Administration (OSHA) was created by Congress to protect people from health and safety risks in the workplace. OSHA sets standards to guard against dangers such as excessive noise and dust, faulty machinery, and toxic fumes. To file a complaint, an employee may obtain the proper form from the federal Division of Industrial Safety, the state OSHA office, or the employer. Employers who do not follow OSHA standards are subject to substantial fines.

The medical insurance specialist should verify a patient's coverage under workers' compensation by contacting the patient's employer and asking for the name of the insurance carrier. Then the carrier should be contacted to find out whether the selected physician is authorized and what information the carrier will need in order to process the claim.

As with other federal health care programs, payment to physicians and other health care providers under FECA is based on the Medicare Fee Schedule. The physician may not bill the patient for more than the allowed charge.

Deadlines for completing the various forms involved in workers' compensation cases are determined by federal law. Bills for medical services must be sent to the OWCP by December 31 of the year following the year in which services were provided, or by December 31 of the year following the year when the condition was first accepted as covered by the workers' compensation program, whichever is later. Generally, of course, bills are submitted promptly by the medical office.

Professional Focus

Workers' Compensation Terminology

The physician's reports in workers' compensation cases use specific terms to describe the job-related effects of certain injuries and disabilities. These terms have been agreed to by state compensation commissions and carriers to create a common understanding of the patient's condition. Here are some examples:

- Levels of pain are described as minimal, slight, moderate, or severe.
- Disability due to heart disease, pulmonary dysfunction, abdominal weakness, or spinal injuries are described in terms of one of the following levels:

  — Limitation to light work.
  — Precluding heavy work.
  — Precluding heavy lifting, repeated bending, and stooping.
  — Precluding heavy lifting.
  —Precluding very heavy work.
  —Precluding very heavy lifting.

- Disability due to lower-extremity injuries are described as either:

  —Limitation to sedentary work.
  —Limitation to semisedentary work.

STATE PROGRAMS, FORMS, AND PROCEDURES

State programs cover traumatic and nontraumatic injuries to state and private business employees within each state, although there are some exceptions. Eligibility and exceptions vary from state to state. A state compensation board or commission administers workers' compensation laws for employees eligible under state laws. These boards or commissions handle employee appeals and provide information to employers and health care providers about regulations.

Determining State Regulations

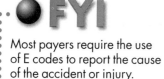

Compliance with state laws is important in workers' compensation cases. Medical insurance specialists should become familiar with the regulations that apply in their states. To learn the law, ask these five important questions of the state compensation board:

1. **What forms and records are required from the medical office, and where can the office get blank forms?**

   Each state has its own system of claim forms and required medical records that must be provided by the physician who treats a person with a job-related injury or illness. The practice should secure the correct forms and comply with filing instructions, deadlines, and rules concerning photocopies and signatures. For example, some states do not accept photocopied signatures, so the physician must sign all photocopies as well as originals.

2. **What organizations and agencies should receive the claim forms, and what are their addresses?**

   Forms and records must be sent to the correct address. Sending information to the wrong place delays processing and reimbursement.

3. **How is reimbursement determined, and can the physician bill the patient or employer for charges in excess of state-determined fees?**

   Reimbursement methods vary from state to state. The state program may use a system of allowed charges or a fee schedule that designates a flat fee for each medical service. It is important to know which method applies and whether excess charges may be billed to the patient or the patient's employer. The physician may be prohibited by law from billing the patient for excess charges.

4. **Who chooses the physician?**

   States may regulate who can choose the treating physician in workers' compensation cases. In some states the patient may choose the physician. In others the physician must be approved by the employer, the insurance carrier, or the state regulatory agency. State programs may not pay for treatment by an unauthorized physician.

   The workers' compensation policies of many insurance carriers require the employer to be in a managed care plan. In this case, the injured employee's claim is overseen by the patient's primary care physician (gatekeeper). This physician is responsible for authorizing the appropriate care needed and for overseeing the employee's claim.

5. **What are the filing deadlines?**

   Filing deadlines must be known and carefully followed. Failure to do so may result in loss of benefits.

General Guidelines for Claims

When a patient is covered by workers' compensation insurance, other insurance plans and programs do not cover the charges or will cover charges only after workers' compensation benefits are exhausted. The medical office specialist files for the patient's workers' compensation benefits through the appropriate insurance carrier. State forms and regulations vary.

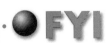
Generally, the physician must complete narrative reports and a claim form. There are no universal rules for completing a claim form. Some plans use the HIPAA 837 or the CMS-1500, while others have their own claim forms. Although the specific procedures vary depending on the state and on the insurance carrier, the following are some general guidelines:

- Payment from the insurance carrier must be accepted as payment in full. Patients or employers may not be billed for any of the medical expenses.
- A separate file must be established when a provider treats an individual who is already a patient of the practice. Information in the patient's regular medical record (nonworkers' compensation) must not be released to the insurance carrier.
- The patient's signature is not required on any billing forms.
- The workers' compensation claim number should be included on all forms and correspondence.
- Use the eight-digit format when reporting dates such as the date last worked.

Employees who become sick or injured due to a work-related incident or environment must report the illness or accident to their employer right away. When this happens, the employer sends a report of occupational illness or injury to the appropriate state office. The employer also typically completes a form that authorizes medical treatment. This form guarantees payment to the treating physician. The injured or ill employee brings it to the physician's office.

After the office visit, the physician prepares a first report of injury or illness. This report must include the following information:

- Dates of examination and treatment
- Patient's history and description of the injury and/or illness as told to the physician
- Name and address of the employer, and name of the employee's supervisor
- Detailed description of the physician's findings
- Results of X-rays and other diagnostic tests
- Diagnosis
- Clinical treatment
- The physician's opinion of the relationship between the work environment and the injury and/or illness, and an explanation of how the physician arrived at that opinion

The first report of injury or illness should be submitted as soon as possible after the office visit. In contrast to usual procedure, this report does not require the patient's signature. The medical insurance specialist sends copies of the report to the state compensation board or commission, the carrier, and the employer; a copy is also filed in a separate work-related medical record for the patient.

When a patient's workers' compensation claim for temporary or permanent disability is accepted by the carrier, the physician continues to monitor the patient's medical condition or disability. The physician is asked to file progress reports (also known as supplemental reports) to explain changes, such as the point in time when an employee with a temporary disability can resume work. In some cases, the patient may receive temporary disability benefits for a period of time while he or she is unable to return to work. Progress reports should include the patient's work status, anticipated additional required treatment, an estimate of future ability to perform occupational tasks, and the extent of permanent loss or disability.

Some states also require a final report from a physician who has completed treatment of a patient covered by workers' compensation.

KEEPING SEPARATE RECORDS

HIPAA Tip

Workers' Compensation and the HIPAA Privacy Rule
Workers' compensation cases provide one of the few situations in which a health care provider may disclose a patient's protected health information to an employer without the patient's authorization. Workers' compensation claim information is not subject to the same confidentiality rules as other medical information.

Explore the Internet

Using your favorite search engine, visit the workers' compensation Web site for your state. What are your state's requirements for workers' compensation coverage? Try to locate a sample claim form for your state. Then locate online newsletters. According to the newsletters, what are some of the current topics in workers' compensation?

Workers' compensation cases are subject to review and court hearings. They usually require medical records in addition to the attending physician's reports and the health care claims. Handling the case and the claim requires information about medical care only for the work-related injury or illness. Records about treatment for other conditions are not needed. In fact, according to law, compensation boards and insurance carriers can review only history and treatment information that pertains to the work-related injury or illness.

When the physician treats a patient with a work-related illness or injury, the medical insurance specialist should set up a separate medical record for the case. This makes pertinent notes and records for the workers' compensation claim easy to find. A signed authorization to release information for the workers' compensation claim should be filed in this separate medical record.

For example, suppose Rachel Goldmeir is seeing Dr. Littlejohn for a back injury she suffered rearranging office furniture during work as an interior designer for Dayton's Interiors. While still in the care of the physician, Ms. Goldmeir seeks care from Dr. Littlejohn for strep throat. The strep throat is not work-related. While the medical office must keep records about the illness, the workers' compensation claims processors do not need these records, nor are they entitled to review them. Therefore, a separate record and ledger for treatment of the back injury must be created. Information about medical care for the strep throat should go in Ms. Goldmeir's regular patient record.

Chapter Summary

1. Workers' compensation insurance covers medical costs, lost wages, and disability benefits for employees with work-related injuries or illnesses. The Office of Workers' Compensation Programs of the U.S. Department of Labor administers the program for civilian federal employees. State compensation boards or commissions administer state programs.

2. Five types of compensation that may be received as workers' compensation benefits are medical treatment, lost wages (temporary disability), permanent disability payments (either partial or full disability), compensation for dependents of employees who are fatally injured, and vocational rehabilitation.

3. Five questions to ask the state compensation board about workers' compensation regulations are:

   - What forms and records are required from the medical office, and where can the office get the blank forms?

   - What organizations and agencies receive information and claim forms, and what are their addresses?

   - How is reimbursement determined, and can the physician bill the patient or employer for charges in excess of state-determined fees?

   - Who chooses the physician?

   - What are the filing deadlines?

4. Medical information related to a workers' compensation case should be filed separately from the patient's regular medical record. Workers' compensation cases are subject to review and court hearings. According to law, organizations and agencies that process the claims may review only history and treatment information that pertains to the work-related injury or illness.

Check Your Understanding

Part 1. Place the letter that corresponds to the term beside the correct definition.

a. FECA
b. final report
c. first report of injury or illness
d. occupational illness
e. OWCP
f. progress report
g. traumatic injury

_____ **1.** A federal law that provides workers' compensation insurance for civilian employees of the federal government.

_____ **2.** A report filed that includes the employer's name and address, the employee's supervisor's name, the dates of examination and treatment, the patient's history and description of what happened, and the physician's diagnosis and opinion of its work-relatedness.

_____ **3.** An injury caused by a specific event or series of events within a single workday or shift.

_____ **4.** The office that administers the Federal Employees' Compensation Act.

_____ **5.** A condition caused by the work environment over a period longer than one workday or shift.

_____ **6.** A report filed by the physician in a workers' compensation case when treatment of the patient's job-related case is finished.

_____ **7.** A report filed by the physician in a workers' compensation case when a patient's medical condition or disability changes.

Part 2. Supply the answers to the following two cases.

A.

Stephen C. Yu hurt his knee while at work. Assume that a first report of injury has been filed and a case number of RB67443 has been issued.

Physician Information:
Name: Lorraine Rutigliano, MD
Employer ID Number: 45-7659871

Patient Information Form:
Name: Stephen C. Yu (New Patient)
Sex: Male
Birth Date: 12-20-69
Address: 12 Baker Road
Springfield, Missouri 65804
Social Security Number: 998-20-8761
Employer: Conrad's Body Shop
70 Bradford Street
Kansas City, Missouri 64590
Phone: 417-660-9988
Insurance Carrier: CIGNA KC (indemnity plan)
Insurance Carrier Address: 60 Twentieth Street
Kansas City, Missouri 64200
Insurance Group Number: G68063

Patient's Encounter Form:
Date: 3-21-2008
Account Number: None
WORKERS' COMPENSATION CASE
PATIENT RECORD NUMBER 665
CC: Patient twisted his knee on Thursday, 3-20-08. Pain is worse on the lateral and inferior aspect of the left knee. No tenderness with active or passive range of motion of the knee.
Dx: Right lateral collateral ligament sprain.

List of Fees for Service:
Charges: Office visit, Level II, $60

Supply the following data elements:

Billing Provider _____

Billing Provider's Primary Identifier _____

Subscriber _____

Patient _____

Relationship _____

Claim Filing Indicator Code _____

Place of Service Code _____

WC Claim Number _____

Payer's Name _____

Payer's ID _____

Diagnosis Codes _____

Total Charge _____

Amount Collected _____

Claim Information

Accident Cause (check one)

   Auto Accident ___ Another Party Responsible ___

   Employment Related ___ Other Accident ___

Date of Accident _____

Service Line Information

Date of Service _____

Procedure Code/Charge _____

Diagnosis Code _____

B.

In the following workers' compensation case, assume that a first report of injury has been filed and that a case number of CA9988 has been issued.

Physician Information:
Name: Dennis L. Pulaski, MD
Employer ID Number: 22-9872767

Patient Information Form:
Name: Myrna Branch Estephan (New Patient)
Sex: Female
Birth Date: April 25, 1947
Address: 346 Austin Boulevard
      San Antonio, Texas 78289
Social Security Number: 968-44-9876
Employer: Consuela's Nail Shop
      644 San Juan Street
      San Antonio, Texas 78299
Phone: 512-681-8674
Insurance Carrier: AETNA TX (PPO)
Insurance Carrier Address: 20 Forester Avenue
      San Antonio, Texas 78287
Insurance Group Number: AR 187267-T

Patient's Encounter Form:
Date: April 22, 2008
Account Number: None
WORKERS' COMPENSATION CASE
PATIENT RECORD NUMBER 56-D
CC: Patient presents for evaluation of left hand numbness that happened today. Nerve conduction studies confirm a left median nerve entrapment at the wrist (carpal tunnel).
Dx: Carpal tunnel syndrome.

List of Fees for Service:
Charges: Office visit; problem-focused history and examination, straightforward decision making (ten-minute appointment), $60
Nerve conduction, amplitude and latency/velocity study, each nerve, all sites along the nerve; sensory, $60

Supply the following data elements:

Billing Provider _____

Billing Provider's Primary Identifier _____

Subscriber _____

Patient _____

Relationship _____

Claim Filing Indicator Code _____

Place of Service Code _____

WC Claim Number _____

Payer's Name _____

Payer's ID _____

Diagnosis Codes _____

Total Charge _____

Amount Collected _____

Claim Information

Accident Cause (check one)

   Auto Accident ___   Another Party Responsible ___

   Employment Related ___   Other Accident ___

Date of Accident _____

Service Line Information

Date of Service _____

Procedure Code/Charge _____

Diagnosis Code _____

Date of Service _____

Procedure Code/Charge _____

Diagnosis Code _____

Objectives

After completing this chapter, you will be able to define the key terms and:

1. Discuss the purpose of disability compensation.
2. Name the six major federal disability programs, and describe who is eligible for program benefits.
3. Compare government and private disability plans.
4. List eight types of information the physician should include in a medical report for the claims department of a disability compensation program.

Key Terms

Civil Service Retirement System (CSRS)

disability compensation programs

Federal Employees Retirement System (FERS)

Federal Insurance Contribution Act (FICA)

Notice of Claim Filed

permanent disability

private disability insurance

prognosis

Social Security Disability Insurance (SSDI)

State Disability Insurance (SDI)

Supplemental Security Income (SSI)

temporary disability

Veteran's Compensation Program

Veteran's Pension Program

Why This Chapter Is Important to You

The information in this chapter will enable you to:

- Be aware of various types of government and private disability compensation programs
- Know what to do when you receive a Notice of Claim Filed from the Social Security Administration
- Help the physician complete requests for medical information for patients who qualify for disability insurance

What Do You Think?

Disability coverage is designed to help people whose ability to work is affected by illness or injury. Many people are covered by their employers' plans or by state disability plans. Other people may purchase private disability coverage. What types of information must the medical office report in disability cases?

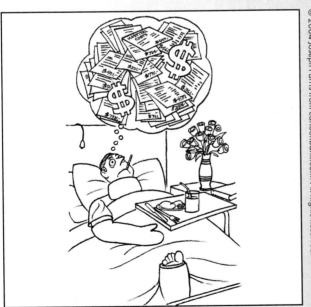

© 2004 Joseph Farris from cartoonbank.com. All Rights Reserved.

Most of the insurance and compensation plans handled by medical insurance specialists are designed to pay for health care costs resulting from illnesses or injuries. By comparison, disability compensation programs pay benefits for lost income when an illness or injury prevents a person from working. Unlike workers' compensation programs, which also include compensation for lost income, the illness or injury does not have to be work-related.

For example, suppose Mark Davidson, who works as a furniture mover, falls down the basement stairs at home and fractures a vertebra in his back. Mark's injury makes it impossible for him to do his job. The amount of cash benefits depends on the extent of Mark's injury and the provisions of the disability compensation program that covers him. The main purpose of most disability compensation programs is to replace wages lost while the person is unable to work.

The federal government, some states, and many private insurance companies offer disability compensation programs and policies. Eligibility and benefits vary. However, they all require the insured to provide convincing medical evidence that the condition resulting from the illness or injury satisfies the criteria given in the program or policy.

Government Disability Programs

There are six major federal disability programs:

- Social Security Disability Insurance (SSDI)
- Supplemental Security Income (SSI)
- Civil Service Retirement System (CSRS)
- Federal Employees Retirement System (FERS)
- Veteran's Compensation Program
- Veteran's Pension Program

People who become disabled may qualify for Social Security Disability Insurance (SSDI) benefits if one of the following applies:

- They are salaried or hourly wage employees whose payroll deductions included those for the Federal Insurance Contribution Act (FICA).

- They are self-employed and paid Social Security taxes for the required minimum number of quarters.

- They are widows, widowers, or minor children of deceased workers who would be qualified for Social Security benefits if they were still alive.

Disability under the SSDI program is defined as a condition that prevents the worker from doing any work and that is expected to last at least twelve consecutive months or can be expected to result in the worker's death. Part of the review process includes an assessment of whether the worker can perform a different job or learn new skills that the condition will allow him or her to use.

The Supplemental Security Income (SSI) program is a welfare program, not an entitlement program. SSI provides payments to individuals in need, including aged, blind, and disabled individuals. Eligibility is determined using nationwide standards.

The Federal Employees Retirement System (FERS) provides disability coverage to federal workers hired after 1984. Employees hired before 1984 enrolled in the Civil Service Retirement System (CSRS). The FERS program consists of a federal disability program and the Social Security disability program. The two parts of the program have different eligibility rules, and some workers qualify for FERS benefits but not for SSDI benefits. If a worker is eligible for both, the amount of the SSDI payment is reduced based on the amount of the FERS payment.

Veterans of the uniformed services are covered by two federal plans, the Veteran's Compensation Program and the Veteran's Pension Program. Certain veterans may qualify to receive benefits from both VA programs. The Veteran's Compensation Program provides coverage for individuals with a permanent and total disability that resulted from a service-related illness or injury. In order for the veteran to be eligible for benefits, the disability must affect his or her earning capacity. The Veteran's Pension Program provides benefits for service-related permanent disability to those who are unable to obtain gainful employment.

In states with disability programs, State Disability Insurance (SDI) covers most workers in the state, although some states list employees of state and federal government, school district employees, and employees of churches as ineligible. As with Social Security Disability Insurance, SDI is usually paid for through payroll deductions.

Private Disability Policies

Individuals can purchase private disability insurance from insurance companies, or a policy may be available to employees through employer-sponsored programs. These plans usually supplement benefits from government programs.

Private plans provide reimbursement for lost income when a disability prevents the injured person from working. They generally recognize two kinds of disabilities. Workers with temporary disabilities cannot do their regular jobs for a short time but are expected to recover completely and return to work. A permanent disability is a condition that prevents the insured worker from returning to the job held before the illness or injury.

FILING FOR DISABILITY BENEFITS

Although medical insurance specialists do not fill out claim forms for disability compensation programs, they may be asked to provide a physician's medical report and accompanying medical records. The physician will need help gathering the information for the report and assembling copies of pertinent records.

Inadequate medical information can result in denial of benefits. When a Notice of Claim Filed is received from Social Security or when another request for medical information is received, the medical insurance specialist works with the physician to document the worker's case. The medical information provided should include evidence of the severity of the illness or injury and how long the physician expects the disability to last. When in doubt, provide more information than appears to be needed rather than not enough.

The disability compensation program may ask the physician to complete a form. Alternatively, the physician may be asked to provide a narrative with the facts and medical opinions that the claim examiner requires. The narrative should include:

- Medical history
- Clinical signs and symptoms
- Diagnosis
- Treatment plan
- Prognosis, that is, the physician's prediction of the outcome of the illness or injury and the likelihood of recovery
- The patient's ability to perform various employment-related functions
- Results of laboratory tests, with copies of laboratory reports
- Other reports as applicable, including hospital history and discharge; audiograms; radiograms; blood tests; biopsies; range-of-motion tests; nuclear medicine tests; pulmonary function tests; and reports from psychologists, social workers, or social service agents.

If the medical narrative prepared for the claim examiner is incomplete, does not contain enough detail, or has errors, the patient may be denied benefits. Therefore, it is very important for the medical insurance specialist to proofread the report for mistakes or missing information before releasing it. In addition, the patient must sign a form to authorize release of information.

Consulting and Educational Career Opportunities

Many new job opportunities are offered in nontraditional environments. The following list describes positions in some of these settings.

- *Pharmaceutical Companies*—The drugs that are tested in clinical trials must be coded for reporting test results to regulatory agencies.
- *Software Development Companies*—A firm that produces a software program for the health care industry requires people who understand claims processing and coding procedures. These employees write the specifications for the program and then test its performance using sample data.
- *Accounting Firms*—Many accounting firms have provider organizations as their clients. The accountants prepare these clients' tax returns and audit their financial records. To assist in this process, they employ professional coders who understand the reimbursement process.
- *Law Firms*—Because of the growing number of lawsuits resulting from fraud and abuse initiatives, many law firms employ—or hire as consultants—both clinical advisers, such as registered nurses, and professional coders and billing specialists who can assist with compliance issues.
- *Independent Consultants*—There are many opportunities for consulting work with provider groups on issues such as compliance plans, preparation of correct forms, and audit procedures.
- *Seminar or Training and Education*—There are numerous opportunities for work as an educator, whether as college faculty or workshop or seminar faculty training physicians and office staff.
- *Contract Work*—Contract work may involve working for a consulting company and being assigned to various client companies (such as on-site coding), or it may involve self-employment as a consultant. Jobs in education may also be as employees or as independent contractors.

Chapter Summary

1. Disability compensation is a government program or an insurance policy designed to reimburse the insured for lost wages caused by an illness or injury.

2. The six major federal disability programs are (a) Social Security Disability Insurance (SSDI), (b) Supplemental Security Income (SSI), (c) Civil Service Retirement System (CSRS), (d) Federal Employees Retirement System (FERS), (e) Veteran's Compensation Program, and (f) Veteran's Pension Program.

The three categories of eligibility for SSDI are (a) salaried or hourly-wage employees whose payroll deductions included those for FICA; (b) self-employed individuals who paid a special Social Security tax; and (c) widows, widowers, or minor children with disabilities whose deceased spouses or parents would qualify for Social Security benefits if they were still alive.

SSI provides cash payments to elderly, blind, and disabled people with incomes below the federal poverty level. CSRS and FERS cover employees of the federal government. The two veteran's programs listed above benefit veterans of the uniformed services.

3. Some government disability programs, such as Social Security Disability Insurance and State Disability Insurance, are funded through employee payroll deductions. Other plans, such as Supplemental Security Income, are welfare programs. Private disability insurance can be purchased or may be available through an employer's plan.

4. Eight types of information the physician should include in a medical report for a disability compensation program are (a) medical history; (b) clinical signs and symptoms; (c) diagnosis; (d) treatment plan; (e) prognosis; (f) the patient's ability to perform various employment-related functions; (g) results of laboratory tests, with copies of laboratory reports; and (h) other reports as applicable.

Part 1. Answer the following questions.

1. What does disability compensation insurance pay for?

_____

2. What are the six major federal disability programs?

_____

3. Which federal disability program is a welfare program?

_____

4. What is the designation of the payroll deduction that pays for the Social Security Disability Insurance program?

_____

5. What is the term used by private disability compensation programs for a condition that prevents a worker from doing a regular job for a short time, but from which the worker is expected to recover?

_____

6. What is the term used by private disability compensation programs for a condition that prevents the insured from returning to the job?

_____

7. What can happen if the claim examiner for a disability compensation program does not have enough medical information?

_____

8. What does the Social Security Administration send the physician when a patient files a claim for disability compensation benefits?

_____

9. What term describes the physician's prediction of the outcome of the illness or injury and the likelihood of recovery?

_____

10. What must a patient sign before medical information can be sent to a claim examiner for a disability compensation program?

_____

Part 2. Analyze the following medical report for a disability compensation program, and identify the major types of information it contains. Select your answers from the following list: clinical signs and symptoms, diagnosis, medical history, prognosis, and treatment plan.

Medical Report on Barry Finestine
Date of Birth: 10-11-50
Date of Examination: 5-07-08
Employer: Marty's Movers, Randolph Road, Forester, NJ 07652

Mr. Finestine came in with a one-month history of back pain with sudden onset from lifting heavy furniture during an office relocation. He complained of pain radiating to his lower left leg to the level of the ankle. Flexion exercises made the condition worse.

_____

Examination of the thoracic lumbar spine reveals flexion to 90 degrees; backward bending is 0 degrees; side bending bilaterally is 30 degrees; rotation bilaterally is 45 degrees. Range of motion of the lumbar spine is full of flexion, extension, lateral bending, and rotation, with some discomfort on extension. Muscle strength, bulk, tone, and light touch are intact. Deep tendon reflexes are two plus over four and symmetric. Toes are down going. Patrick's test is negative bilaterally. There is mild joint tenderness and mild left sciatic notch tenderness. Spring test is negative.

---

(1) Thoracic lumbar strain.

(2) Acute low-back pain with radicular pain into the left leg without neurologic evidence of radiculopathy.

(3) Probable chronic lumbar myositis.

---

(1) Bed rest with local heat for twenty-four hours.

(2) Flexion exercises, adding extension exercises as he improves.

(3) Prednisone two milligrams TID with meals and Tylenol #3 if needed for pain control.

Patient follow-up scheduled for one week.

Discussed with the patient need to avoid heavy lifting for the next three months.

Part 3. Study the following draft of a letter from a physician in response to a Notice of Claim Filed. Assume the role of the medical insurance specialist in this situation. In your opinion, are there any elements missing from this letter that should be included?

---

re: ROGER MONTOYA

At home on the basement stairs, Mr. Montoya fell and injured his right wrist and right knee on January 2, 2008. The right wrist is swollen and has an obvious deformity. There is normal sensation and normal motion of fingers. He reports pain with movement of the wrist. Right knee patella is tender to palpitation. There is joint effusion of the knee.

An X-ray of the right wrist shows distal radial fracture. Right knee X-ray shows a fracture of the patella with no displacement of the fragments.

My diagnosis is: Colles fracture, right wrist, and patellar fracture, right knee.

I have immobilized the right leg. Mr. Montoya has been supplied with one crutch and instructed in crutch walking. He has been told to put as little weight as possible on the knee. He should not perform his normal work at Majors' Delicatessen.

CHAPTER 14 Dental Insurance

Objectives

After completing this chapter, you will be able to define the key terms and:

1. Locate and describe the parts of the mouth and the teeth.
2. Recognize key words, conditions, and treatments related to dentistry.
3. Describe six types of benefits offered by dental insurance plans.
4. Discuss the claim form and coding methods commonly used to submit dental insurance claims.

Key Terms

ADA Dental Claim Form

canines

Current Dental Terminology
  (CDT-4)

dentin

Dentist's Pretreatment
  Estimate

Dentist's Statement of Actual
  Services

enamel

gingivae (*sing.*, gingiva)

incisors

mandible

maxilla

maxillofacial surgery

molars

occlusion

oral cavity

oral surgery

palate

premolars

prophylaxes (*sing.*,
  prophylaxis)

prostheses (*sing.*, prosthesis)

pulp

uvula

Why This Chapter Is Important to You

The information in this chapter will enable you to:

- Understand the language that dentists use to describe diagnoses and procedures.
- Help patients with dental insurance claims.

What Do You Think?

Some insurance specialists work in dental practices, rather than in medical practices. How might the tasks or surroundings of a dental insurance specialist be different from those of a medical insurance specialist?

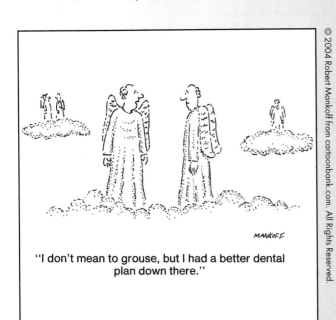

"I don't mean to grouse, but I had a better dental plan down there."

INTRODUCTION TO DENTAL TERMS

Medical terminology is used to describe oral (related to the mouth) anatomy, diagnoses, and treatments. In dentistry, the word elements of roots, combining vowels, prefixes, and suffixes are put together to describe the specific parts of the mouth and teeth as well as the procedures performed.

Overview of the Parts of the Mouth and the Teeth

The mouth, shown in Figure 14-1, is at the beginning of the digestive system. It has an outer part, made up of the lips and cheeks, and an inner section, or oral cavity, leading to the throat. The oral cavity contains the gums, called gingivae; the teeth; the tongue; and the tonsils.

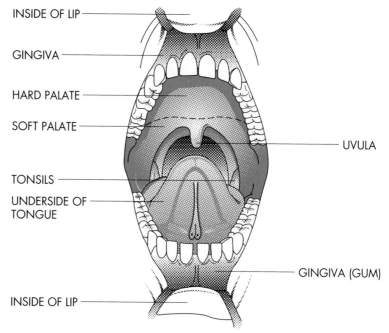

Figure 14-1 The Mouth

The mouth's underlying bone structure also has two major parts. The mandible, the U-shaped lower jawbone, has tooth sockets to hold the lower teeth. The upper jawbone is the maxilla. It houses the upper teeth and the palate, which is the roof of the mouth. The hard palate is a bony structure that separates the oral cavity from the inner nose, or nasal cavity. The soft palate, made up of muscle tissue, is located behind the hard palate. The soft palate extends downward toward the throat, ending in the cone-shaped uvula. The upper and lower jawbones are connected by a joint. When the jaws close, the contact between the upper and lower teeth is referred to as occlusion.

The teeth tear and grind food, which is moistened by saliva from the salivary glands. Saliva not only helps to soften food; it also contains an enzyme that begins the breakdown, or digestion, of food. When a person swallows, muscles pull the soft palate and uvula upward, closing the opening between the nasal cavity and the pharynx. This keeps food from entering the nasal cavity.

The thirty-two permanent teeth that adults have are set in two arches, one in the mandible and the other in the maxilla. Each of the jaws holds four incisors, which are the cutting teeth; two canines; four premolars; and six molars. In dental insurance claims, the teeth are numbered from a person's right to left, upper to lower, as shown in Figure 14-2.

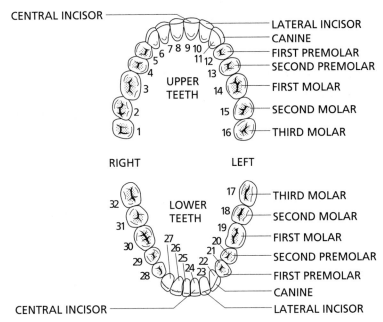

Figure 14–2 The Teeth

Figure 14-3 shows the structure of a tooth. The teeth are held in their sockets by periodontal ligaments. Each tooth is covered by an outer coating, the enamel. A hard material called dentin fills up 80 to 90 percent of the tooth, covering the soft core, or pulp, which contains nerves and blood vessels.

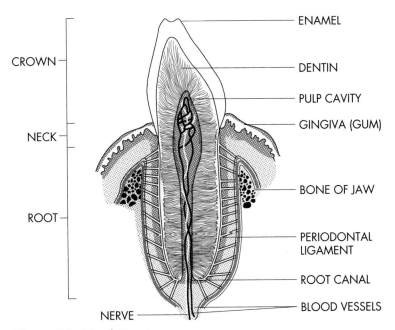

Figure 14–3 Tooth Structure

A tooth has three main sections: the crown, the neck, and the root. The cavity that contains the pulp is called the root canal. The part that is covered with enamel is the crown. The neck is the section where the tooth meets the gum. The section below the gum line is the root.

Examples of dental terms used in dental practices are:

Term	Meaning
Endodontics	Branch of dentistry dealing with tooth pulp
Gingivitis	Inflammation of the gingiva(e)
Malocclusion	Poor alignment of upper and lower teeth
Orthodontics	Branch of dentistry dealing with the correction and prevention of irregular teeth and malocclusion
Periodontics	Branch of dentistry that studies the tissues around the teeth
Periodontitis	Gum disease

DENTAL INSURANCE

As with medical insurance, a broad range of dental insurance plans can be purchased by individuals or by employers. More than 170 million people in the United States have some form of dental insurance. Most insurance carriers' dental plans reimburse policyholders, or subscribers, for dental expenses. However, some carriers offer managed care plans for dental benefits. Currently, about one-third of those insured are covered by some form of managed care for dental insurance. Also, as with medical insurance, participating dentists accept assignment; nonparticipating dentists are paid specific listed fees.

Dental benefits vary. Some of the plans include:

- Preventive Benefits—These benefits cover prophylaxes, or cleanings, at regular intervals and the application of fluoride treatments to coat the teeth of children.

- Diagnostic Benefits—Diagnostic procedures, such as X-rays and laboratory work, are used by the dentist to evaluate conditions and determine what dental treatment is needed.

- Basic Benefits—In most plans, these benefits cover restorative work such as fillings, crowns, and inlays; endodontic procedures such as root canal fillings; and periodontic procedures to prevent or treat gum disease.

- Prosthodontics Benefits—These benefits cover the construction of bridges and dentures, called dental prostheses, and the repair of existing prosthetic appliances. Most dental contracts limit the number and timing of prosthesis replacements.

- Orthodontic Benefits—These benefits cover the use of braces and other devices to straighten teeth.

- Oral and Maxillofacial Surgery—Oral surgery and maxillofacial surgery (surgical procedures relating to the face and jaw) as well as the necessary general anesthesia are covered.

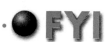

FYI

Many dental plans cover routine periodic examinations. For example, some plans cover a routine examination every six months. In order for insurance to cover the charge, the interval between appointments must be no less than six months and one day. For instance, appointments on March 3 and September 3 would be considered two visits in six months, and the second visit would not be covered.

Carriers do not normally pay the same percentage for every type of procedure. For example, many plans cover the cost of prophylaxes and examinations in full, but they may pick up only 50 to 90 percent of other procedures.

Medicare offers no dental coverage. However, it does cover oral surgery procedures for conditions such as tumors or jaw disease under its medical benefits. Some dental procedures are covered under Medicaid; the fees are set by the individual states. Most Blue Cross and Blue Shield plans include dental coverage contracts.

PROCESSING DENTAL CLAIMS

Dental patients complete patient information forms similar to those used in medical offices. The patient provides personal and employment information, dental insurance information, and account information. The dental patient information form usually has a signature line for authorization of release of information. The patient's encounter form, too, is similar to that used in medical offices. An example is shown in Figure 14-4 on page 217.

Dental Coding

In general, dental insurance claims require procedure codes, but not diagnosis codes. Surgical procedures submitted on a medical claim form are the exception. In these cases, diagnosis codes are also required. Dental procedure codes are five-digit codes that begin with the letter D to make them different from numbers in other coding systems. The second number of the code indicates the category of dental service. There are twelve categories:

Category of Service	Code Series
I. Diagnostic	D0100–D0999
II. Preventive	D1000–D1999
III. Restorative	D2000–D2999
IV. Endodontics	D3000–D3999
V. Periodontics	D4000–D4999
VI. Prosthodontics, Removable	D5000–D5899
VII. Maxillofacial Prosthetics	D5900–D5999
VIII. Implant Services	D6000–D6199
IX. Prosthodontics, Fixed	D6200–D6999
X. Oral and Maxillofacial Surgery	D7000–D7999
XI. Orthodontics	D8000–D8999
XII. Adjunctive General Services	D9000–D9999

The American Dental Association (ADA) develops and maintains the dental codes. They were most recently updated in 2002 in a publication entitled *Current Dental Terminology*, Fourth Edition. The codes are referred to as the CDT-4 codes. The diagnosis codes for claims involving oral surgery or maxillofacial surgery are usually taken from the ICD-9.

Case Study 14-1

Procedure: Performed root canal filling on Tooth 18.

Procedure code (refer to Figure 14-4):

_____

Case Study 14-2

Procedure: Established patient Toru Hayashi complained of pain in the upper or lower right area during his annual checkup. Two bitewings (X-rays designed to show the crowns of the upper and lower teeth at the same time) were taken of the area. Indicated requirement for filling; appointment made for March 22.

Procedure codes (refer to Figure 14-4):

_____

Michael Davis, DDS

Provider: _____

_____

ID #: _____ Tax ID: _____

Name: _____

Address: _____

_____

Pat#: _____ Document: 8889

Code: _____ Date: 09-09-2008

Phone: _____ Time: _____

Codes	— Services —
D0120	PERIODIC ORAL EVALUATION
D0140	LIMITED ORAL EVALUATION - PROBLEM FOCUSED
D1203	FLUORIDE-TOPICAL CHILD (PROPHY NOT INCLUDED)
D1351	SEALANT, PER TOOTH
D2140	AMAL 1 SURF PRIMARY OR PERM
D2330	RESIN-BASED COMP 1 SURFACE ANTERIOR
D2530	INLAY METALLIC - THREE SURF OR MORE
D2750	PORC CRN FUSED TO HIGH NOBLE METAL
D2751	PORC CRN FUSED TO PREDOMINATELY BASE METAL
D2790	FULL CAST CROWN HIGH NOBLE METAL
D2920	RECMT CROWN
D2930	PREFAB. SS CROWN - PRIMARY TOOTH
D2932	PREFAB. RESIN CROWN
D2940	SEDATIVE FILLING
D2950	CORE BUILDUPS INCLUDING ANY PINS
D2952	CAST POST & CORE/ADD. TO CR.
D3110	PULP CAP DIRECT (EXCLUDING FINAL RESTORATION)
D3320	ROOT CANAL, BICUSPID (EXCLUDING FINAL RESTORATION)
D3330	ROOT CANAL, MOLARI (EXCLUDING FINAL RESTORATION)
D5110	COMP DENTURE—MAXILLARY
D5130	IMMEDIATE DENTURE—MAXILLARY
D5213	PARTIAL DENTURE—MAXILLARY
D5214	PARTIAL DENTURE—MANDIBULAR
D5710	REBASE COMP MAXILLARY DENTURE
D5750	RELINE COMP MAXILLARY DENTURE
D5751	RELINE COMP MANDIBULAR DENTURE
D6750	FIXED PARTIAL DENTURE (RETAINER) CROWN: PORCELAIN FUSED TO HIGH NOBLE METAL
D6790	FIXED PARTIAL DENTURE (RETAINER) CROWN: FULL CAST HIGH NOBLE METAL
D6950	PRECISION ATTACHMENT
D7111	EXTRACTION: CORONAL REMNANTS
D9940	OCCLUSAL GUARD, BY REPORT

Description: _____

Codes	— X Rays —
D0272	BITEWINGS 2 FILMS
D0274	BITEWINGS 4 FILMS

Codes	— Payments —
PMTDUE	PAYMENT DUE
CASH	CASH PAYMENT—THANK YOU!
CHECK	CHECK—THANK YOU!
MO	Money Order Payment—Thank You

Family Aging Balances

Current	30	60	90
_____	_____	_____	_____

Remarks: _____

Next Appointment: _____

Previous Balance _____

Today's Charges _____

Amount Paid _____

New Balance _____

Figure 14–4 Dental Office Encounter Form

Dental Claim Forms

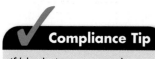

Compliance Tip

If blank 4 is answered yes, blanks 5 through 11 should be completed. The information in blanks 5 through 11 is used to determine which other carriers, if any, have primary liability for the provided treatment.

A dental claim form is used for two purposes: (1) to report the Dentist's Pretreatment Estimate to an insurance carrier before the service is performed, for an analysis of what will be reimbursed, and (2) to submit the Dentist's Statement of Actual Services for claim processing and payment.

A Dentist's Pretreatment Estimate may be submitted for a number of reasons. The primary reason is to find out whether the procedure is covered and the amount of the reimbursement. In addition, this estimate helps to resolve the disagreements that at times arise between a dentist and a carrier about appropriate treatments. Also, dental patients often have choices regarding treatments. For example, one type of crown material may look better than another, but it may also be more expensive. If the dental insurance coverage has a set rate for a crown, a patient who desires the more expensive material may have to pay a higher cost.

Some dental office staff process claims for patients or may offer the patient help with completing claims. Many dental practitioners complete a universal claim form called the ADA Dental Claim Form for patients to attach to their own carriers' claim forms. The ADA Dental Claim Form is approved and updated by the American Dental Association (see Figures 14-5a and b). This form contains eleven sections. The top portion contains patient coverage information, the middle portion contains details about the examination and treatment plan, and the lower portion contains information on authorizations and billing details, such as the billing dentist.

When treatment involves a medical claim for oral or maxillofacial surgery, the claim must be submitted using the electronic HIPAA claim or the CMS-1500 paper claim form, depending on the carrier. The state Medicare carrier has specific guidelines for using the electronic HIPAA claim.

Filling Out the ADA Dental Claim Form

The instructions for completing the ADA Dental Claim Form are similar to those for other claims. Step-by-step instructions on how to fill in each blank on the form appear on the back of the form and are shown in Figure 14-5b on page 220.

Explore the Internet

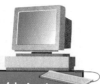

Visit the Web site of the American Dental Association. Go to the A-Z topics section in the panel entitled Your Oral Health, and research the topic of insurance. What types of dental plans are available today?

ADA Dental Claim Form

HEADER INFORMATION

1. Type of Transaction (Check all applicable boxes)

☐ Statement of Actual Services – OR – ☐ Request for Predetermination / Preauthorization

☐ EPSDT / Title XIX

2. Predetermination / Preauthorization Number

PRIMARY PAYER INFORMATION

3. Name, Address, City, State, Zip Code

OTHER COVERAGE

4. Other Dental or Medical Coverage? ☐ No (Skip 5-11) ☐ Yes (Complete 5-11)

5. Subscriber Name (Last, First, Middle Initial, Suffix)

6. Date of Birth (MM/DD/CCYY)	7. Gender ☐ M ☐ F	8. Subscriber Identifier (SSN or ID#)

9. Plan/Group Number	10. Relationship to Primary Subscriber (Check applicable box) ☐ Self ☐ Spouse ☐ Dependent ☐ Other

11. Other Carrier Name, Address, City, State, Zip Code

PRIMARY SUBSCRIBER INFORMATION

12. Name (Last, First, Middle Initial, Suffix), Address, City, State, Zip Code

13. Date of Birth (MM/DD/CCYY)	14. Gender ☐ M ☐ F	15. Subscriber Identifier (SSN or ID#)

16. Plan/Group Number	17. Employer Name

PATIENT INFORMATION

18. Relationship to Primary Subscriber (Check applicable box) ☐ Self ☐ Spouse ☐ Dependent Child ☐ Other   19. Student Status ☐ FTS ☐ PTS

20. Name (Last, First, Middle Initial, Suffix), Address, City, State, Zip Code

21. Date of Birth (MM/DD/CCYY)	22. Gender ☐ M ☐ F	23. Patient ID/Account # (Assigned by Dentist)

RECORD OF SERVICES PROVIDED

	24. Procedure Date (MM/DD/CCYY)	25. Area of Oral Cavity	26. Tooth System	27. Tooth Number(s) or Letter(s)	28. Tooth Surface	29. Procedure Code	30. Description	31. Fee
1								
2								
3								
4								
5								
6								
7								
8								
9								
10								

MISSING TEETH INFORMATION

34. (Place an 'X' on each missing tooth)

Permanent																Primary									
1	2	3	4	5	6	7	8	9	10	11	12	13	14	15	16	A	B	C	D	E	F	G	H	I	J
32	31	30	29	28	27	26	25	24	23	22	21	20	19	18	17	T	S	R	Q	P	O	N	M	L	K

32. Other Fee(s)

33. Total Fee

35. Remarks

AUTHORIZATIONS

36. I have been informed of the treatment plan and associated fees. I agree to be responsible for all charges for dental services and materials not paid by my dental benefit plan, unless prohibited by law, or the treating dentist or dental practice has a contractual agreement with my plan prohibiting all or a portion of such charges. To the extent permitted by law, I consent to your use and disclosure of my protected health information to carry out payment activities in connection with this claim.

X_____

Patient/Guardian signature   Date

37. I hereby authorize and direct payment of the dental benefits otherwise payable to me, directly to the below named dentist or dental entity.

X_____

Subscriber signature   Date

ANCILLARY CLAIM/TREATMENT INFORMATION

38. Place of Treatment (Check applicable box) ☐ Provider's Office ☐ Hospital ☐ ECF ☐ Other

39. Number of Enclosures (00 to 99) Radiograph(s) Oral Image(s) Model(s)

40. Is Treatment for Orthodontics? ☐ No (Skip 41-42) ☐ Yes (Complete 41-42)

41. Date Appliance Placed (MM/DD/CCYY)

42. Months of Treatment Remaining

43. Replacement of Prosthesis? ☐ No ☐ Yes (Complete 44)

44. Date Prior Placement (MM/DD/CCYY)

45. Treatment Resulting from (Check applicable box) ☐ Occupational illness/injury ☐ Auto accident ☐ Other accident

46. Date of Accident (MM/DD/CCYY)

47. Auto Accident State

BILLING DENTIST OR DENTAL ENTITY (Leave blank if dentist or dental entity is not submitting claim on behalf of the patient or insured/subscriber)

48. Name, Address, City, State, Zip Code

49. Provider ID	50. License Number	51. SSN or TIN

52. Phone Number ( ) —

TREATING DENTIST AND TREATMENT LOCATION INFORMATION

53. I hereby certify that the procedures as indicated by date are in progress (for procedures that require multiple visits) or have been completed and that the fees submitted are the actual fees I have charged and intend to collect for those procedures.

X_____

Signed (Treating Dentist)   Date

54. Provider ID	55. License Number

56. Address, City, State, Zip Code

57. Phone Number ( ) —	58. Treating Provider Specialty

©**American Dental Association, 2002**
J515 (Same as ADA Dental Claim Form) – J516, J517, J518, J519

To Reorder call 1-800-947-4746
or go online at www.adacatalog.org

Figure 14–5a Front of ADA Dental Claim Form

The form is designed so that the Primary Payer's name and address (Item 3) is visible in a standard #10 window envelope. Please fold the form using the 'tick-marks' printed in the left and right margins. The upper-right blank space is provided for insertion of the third-party payer's claim or control number.

a)   All data elements are required unless noted to the contrary on the face of the form, or in the Data Element Specific Instructions that follow.
b)   When a name and address field is required, the full entity or individual name, address, and Zip code must be entered (i.e., Items 3, 11, 12, 20 and 48).
c)   All dates must include the four-digit year (i.e., Items 6, 13, 21, 24, 36, 37, 41, 44, and 53).
d)   If the number of procedures being reported exceeds the number of lines available on one claim form, the remaining procedures must be listed on a separate, fully completed claim form. Both claim forms are submitted to the third-party payer.

Data Element Specific Instructions

1.   **EPSDT / Title XIX** -- Mark box if patient is covered by state Medicaid's **E**arly and **P**eriodic **S**creening, **D**iagnosis and **T**reatment program for persons under age 21.
2.   Enter number provided by the payer when submitting a claim for services that have been predetermined or preauthorized.
4-11. Leave blank if no other coverage.
8.   The subscriber's Social Security Number (SSN) or other identifier (ID#) assigned by the payer.
15. The subscriber's Social Security Number (SSN) or other identifier (ID#) assigned by the payer.
16. Subscriber's or employer group's Plan or Policy Number. May also be known as the Certificate Number. [Not the subscriber's identification number.]
19-23. Complete only if the patient is **not** the Primary Subscriber. (i.e., "Self" not checked in Item 18)
19. Check "FTS" if patient is a dependent and full-time student; "PTS" if a part-time student. Otherwise, leave blank.
23. Enter if dentist's office assigns a unique number to identify the patient that is **not** the same as the Subscriber Identifier number assigned by the payer (e.g., Chart #).
25. Designate tooth number or letter when procedure code directly involves a tooth. Use area of the oral cavity code set from ANSI/ADA/ISO Specification No. 3950 'Designation System for Teeth and Areas of the Oral Cavity'.
26. Enter applicable ANSI ASC X12 code list qualifier: Use "**JP**" when designating teeth using the ADA's Universal/National Tooth Designation System. Use "**JO**" when using the ANSI/ADA/ISO Specification No. 3950.
27. Designate tooth number when procedure code reported directly involves a tooth. If a range of teeth is being reported, use a hyphen ('-') to separate the first and last tooth in the range. Commas are used to separate individual tooth numbers or ranges applicable to the procedure code reported.
28. Designate tooth surface(s) when procedure code reported directly involves one or more tooth surfaces. Enter up to five of the following codes, without spaces: **B** = Buccal; **D** = Distal; **F** = Facial; **L** = Lingual; **M** = Mesial; and **O** = Occlusal.
29. Use appropriate dental procedure code from current version of *Code on Dental Procedures and Nomenclature*.
31. Dentist's full fee for the dental procedure reported.
32. Used when other fees applicable to dental services provided must be recorded. Such fees include state taxes, where applicable, and other fees imposed by regulatory bodies.
33. Total of all fees listed on the claim form.
34. Report missing teeth on each claim submission.
35. Use "Remarks" space for additional information such as 'reports' for '999' codes or multiple supernumerary teeth.
36. Patient Signature: The patient is defined as an individual who has established a professional relationship with the dentist for the delivery of dental health care. For matters relating to communication of information and consent, this term includes the patient's parent, caretaker, guardian, or other individual as appropriate under state law and the circumstances of the case.
37. Subscriber Signature: Necessary when the patient/insured and dentist wish to have benefits paid directly to the provider. This is an authorization of payment. It does not create a contractual relationship between the dentist and the payer.
38. ECF is the acronym for **E**xtended **C**are **F**acility (e.g., nursing home).
48-52. Leave blank if dentist or dental entity is **not** submitting claim on behalf of the patient or insured/subscriber.
48. The individual dentist's name or the name of the group practice/corporation responsible for billing and other pertinent information. This may differ from the actual treating dentist's name. This is the information that should appear on any payments or correspondence that will be remitted to the billing dentist.
49. Identifier assigned to Billing Dentist of Dental Entity other than the SSN or TIN. Necessary when assigned by carrier receiving the claim
50. Refers to the license number of the billing dentist. This may differ from that of the treating (rendering) dentist that appears in the treating dentist's signature block.
52. The Internal Revenue Service requires that either the Social Security Number (SSN) or Tax Identification Number (TIN) of the billing dentist or dental entity be supplied **only** if the provider accepts payment directly from the third-party payer.
     When the payment is being accepted directly report the: 1) SSN if the billing dentist in unincorporated; 2) Corporation TIN if the billing dentist is incorporated; or 3) Entity TIN when the billing entity is a group practice or clinic.
53. The treating, or rendering, dentist's signature and date the claim form was signed. Dentists should be aware that they have ethical and legal obligations to refund fees for services that are paid in advance but not completed.
56. Full address, including city, state and zip code, where treatment performed by treating (rendering) dentist.
58. Enter the code that indicates the type of dental professional rendering the service from the 'Dental Service Providers' section of the *Healthcare Providers Taxonomy* code list. The current list is posted at: http://www.wpc-edi.com/codes/codes.asp. The available taxonomy codes, as of the first printing of this claim form, follow printed in **boldface**.

122300000X Dentist -- A dentist is a person qualified by a doctorate in dental surgery (D.D.S.) or dental medicine (D.M.D.) licensed by the state to practice dentistry, and practicing within the scope of that license.

Many dentists are general practitioners who handle a wide variety of dental needs.
1223G0001X   General Practice

Other dentists practice in one of nine specialty areas recognized by the American Dental Association:
1223D0001X Dental Public Health
1223E0200X Endodontics
1223P0106X Oral & Maxillofacial Pathology
1223D0008X Oral and Maxillofacial Radiology
1223S0112X Oral & Maxillofacial Surgery
1223X0400X Orthodontics
1223P0221X Pediatric Dentistry
        (Pedodontics)
1223P0300X Periodontics
1223P0700X Prosthodontics

Figure 14-5b Back of ADA Dental Claim Form

Chapter Summary

1. The major parts of the mouth are the lips, cheeks, teeth, gums, tongue, palate, and throat. Each tooth has an outer coating, the enamel; a core, called the dentin; and pulp, containing the nerves and blood supply. The main sections of a tooth are the crown, the neck, and the root.

2. Many dental terms are based on anatomy. For example, the word *malocclusion* means a condition of poor alignment of the upper and lower teeth.

3. The six types of dental benefits offered by dental insurance plans are preventive, diagnostic, basic, prosthodontic, orthodontic, and those for oral and maxillofacial surgeries.

4. The procedures shown on dental insurance claims are coded with CDT-4 codes. Unless the claim is for oral or maxillofacial surgery, ICD-9 diagnosis codes are not required. The universal dental claim form approved by the American Dental Association is called the ADA Dental Claim Form. In dentistry, the electronic HIPPA claim or the CMS-1500 paper claim form is used only to report medical claims for oral and maxillofacial surgeries.

Check Your Understanding

Part 1. Choose the best answer.

_____ **1.** The maxilla is the:
   a. upper jawbone
   b. lower jawbone
   c. joint connecting the upper and lower jawbones

_____ **2.** The gingivae are the:
   a. contacts between upper and lower teeth
   b. gums
   c. incisors

_____ **3.** On a dental claim form, a treated tooth is indicated by:
   a. the name of the tooth
   b. the letter of the tooth
   c. the number of the tooth

_____ **4.** A regular cleaning of the teeth by a dentist to prevent disease is called:
   a. prosthesis
   b. prophylaxis
   c. impaction

_____ **5.** A set of dentures is a:
   a. prosthesis
   b. prophylaxis
   c. impaction

_____ **6.** In general, claims for dental treatments require:
   a. diagnosis codes
   b. procedure codes
   c. neither a nor b

_____ **7.** CDT codes begin with:
   a. a C
   b. an R
   c. a D

_____ **8.** Claims for oral surgery are reported on the:
   a. HIPAA or CMS-1500 form
   b. ADA form
   c. CMS-1450 form

_____ **9.** A dental claim form may be submitted for:
   a. a pretreatment estimate
   b. payment
   c. both a and b

_____**10.** When completing a dental claim form for a dental treatment:
   a. indicate treatments due to illness, injury, or accidents
   b. complete the deductible and maximum allowable blanks
   c. be sure the office manager signs the form

Part 2. Using the most recent CDT-4 available, complete the following case studies. (If you do not have access to the CDT-4, ask your instructor for a list of dental procedure codes.)

1. Procedure: Patient Sarah Rabinowitz, age eight; first examination.

   Code: _____

2. Procedure: 3-20-2008, patient Rory Wetsell, two-surface amalgam/filling on Tooth 15, permanent tooth; local anesthesia.

   Codes: _____

Part 3. Identify the number of the form locator(s) on the ADA Dental Claim Form where the following data should be entered.

____ 1. Blue Cross and Blue Shield claim

____ 2. The fact that the patient has another dental plan

____ 3. The insured's date of birth when the insured is not the patient

____ 4. The name of the dental practice or dentist responsible for generating the charges shown on the claim

____ 5. Date of prior placement of a prosthesis

Part 4. Enter the correct CDT-4 code for each of the following procedures or services.

____ 1. Pulp vitality tests

____ 2. Prophylaxis–child

____ 3. Surgical incision to remove a foreign body from skin

____ 4. Extraction of coronal remnants

____ 5. Inlay—resin-based composite—three surfaces

____ 6. Nasal prosthesis

____ 7. Repair missing teeth in complete dentures

____ 8. Gingivectomy or gingivoplasty—four contiguous teeth per quadrant

____ 9. Endodontic therapy of molar (without final restoration)

____ 10. Recement crown

CHAPTER 15

Hospital Insurance

Objectives

After completing this chapter, you will be able to define the key terms and:

1. Compare inpatient and outpatient hospital services.
2. List the major steps relating to hospital claims processing.
3. Describe two differences in coding diagnoses for hospital inpatient cases and physician office services.
4. Describe the procedure codes used in hospital coding.
5. Discuss the important items that are reported on the HIPAA hospital claim, the 8371.

Key Terms

admitting diagnosis
ambulatory care
attending physician
charge master
charge ticket
CMS-1450
diagnosis-related group
   (DRG)

8371
emergency care
health information
   management (HIM)
inpatient
master patient index

principal diagnosis
principal procedure
Prospective Payment System
   (PPS)
registration
UB-92

Why This Chapter Is Important to You

The information in this chapter will enable you to:

- Become familiar with the coding systems used in hospitals
- Learn the basic billing process that hospitals follow
- Understand the format and use of the UB-92 claim form

What Do You Think?

There are many working and financial agreements between physicians and hospitals; physicians in practices may have staff privileges at hospitals or be associated with hospitals as medical specialists. Medical insurance specialists often prepare claims for surgery and other procedures performed by the physicians who employ them. Why do you think it is important to be aware of the coding systems and the billing process used in hospitals?

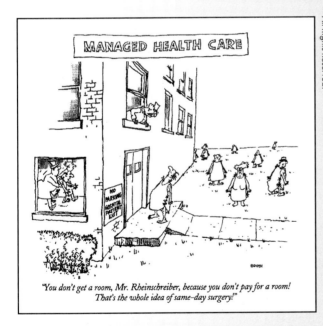

"You don't get a room, Mr. Rheinschreiber, because you don't pay for a room! That's the whole idea of same-day surgery!"

HEALTH CARE FACILITIES: INPATIENT VERSUS OUTPATIENT

General hospitals accept all types of patients. Specialized health care hospitals offer services such as acute care, psychiatric care, and rehabilitation. Private hospitals are either for-profit, investor-owned institutions or nonprofit facilities. Public hospitals are those owned by the federal government (such as veterans' and military hospitals), by states (such as long-term psychiatric facilities and teaching hospitals), and by local governments such as counties and cities. The sizes of hospitals, measured by the number of beds, vary from small to very large.

Inpatient Care

Inpatient facilities are equipped for patients to stay overnight. In addition to hospital admission, inpatient care may be provided in:

- Skilled Nursing Facilities (SNF)—Facilities that provide skilled nursing or rehabilitation services to help with recovery after a hospital stay. Skilled nursing care includes care given by licensed nurses under the direction of a physician, such as intravenous injections, tube feeding, and changing sterile dressings on a wound.

- Long-Term Care Facilities—This term describes facilities such as nursing homes that provide care for patients with chronic disabilities and prolonged illnesses.

- Hospital Emergency Rooms or Departments—Emergency care involves a situation in which a delay in the treatment of the patient would lead to a significant increase in the threat to life or a body part. Emergency care differs from urgently needed care, in which the condition must be treated right away but is not life-threatening.

Outpatient or Ambulatory Care

Many hospitals have expanded beyond inpatient services to offer a variety of outpatient settings. Outpatient care, often called ambulatory care, covers all types of health services that do not require an overnight hospital stay, such as same-day surgery. Most hospitals, for example, have outpatient departments that provide these services.

Different types of outpatient services are also provided in patients' home settings. Home health care services include care given at home, such as physical therapy or skilled nursing care. Home health care is provided by a home health agency (HHA), an organization that provides home care services, including skilled nursing care, physical therapy, occupational therapy, speech therapy, and care by home health aides. At-home recovery care is a different category that includes help with the activities of daily living (ADLs), such as bathing and eating. Hospice care is a special approach to caring for people with terminal illnesses in a familiar and comfortable place, either a special hospice facility or the patient's home.

HOSPITAL CLAIMS PROCESSING

Hospitals generally have large departments that are responsible for major business functions. The admissions department records the patient's personal and financial information. As in medical offices, hospital admissions staff must be sure patients give written consent for the work to be done and for the claim reporting that follows. The patient accounting department handles billing, and there is often a separate collections department. Organizing and maintaining patient medical records in hospitals are the duties of the health information management (HIM) department. Hospitals are also structured into departments for patient care. For example, there are professional services departments, such as laboratory, radiology, and surgery, as well as support services departments, such as food service and housekeeping.

From the insurance perspective, the three major steps in a patient's hospital stay are:

1. Admission, for creating or updating the patient's medical record, verifying patient insurance coverage, securing consent for release of information to payers, and collecting advance payments as appropriate.
2. Treatment, during which the various departments' services are provided and charges generated.
3. Discharge from the hospital or transfer to another facility, at which point the patient's record is compiled, claims or bills are created, and payment is followed up.

Admission

Patients are admitted to hospitals in a process called registration. Like physician practices, hospitals must keep clear, accurate records of their patients' diagnoses and treatments. The record begins at a patient's first admission to the facility. More information is gathered for a hospital admission than is required for a visit to a physician practice. Special points about the patient's care, such as language requirements, religion, or disabilities, are also entered in the record.

CMS requires hospitals to give Medicare patients a copy of the one-page printout entitled "An Important Message from Medicare" on registration. The printout explains the beneficiary's rights as a hospital patient as well as his or her appeal rights regarding hospital discharge (see Figure 15-1 on page 228).

The HIM department keeps a health record system that permits storage and retrieval of clinical information by patient name or number, by attending physician (the physician who is primarily responsible for the care of the patient during the hospital stay), and by diagnosis and procedure. At almost every facility, a part or all of the records are stored in a computer system. Each patient is listed in a patient register under a unique number. These numbers make up the master patient index—the main database that identifies patients.

Outpatient department and emergency room insurance claims are often delayed because it is difficult to verify insurance coverage in these settings. The emergency department has its own registration system because people who come for emergency and urgent treatment must receive care immediately.

IMPORTANT MESSAGE FROM MEDICARE

YOUR RIGHTS AS A HOSPITAL PATIENT

- You have the right to receive necessary hospital services covered by Medicare, or covered by your Medicare Health Plan ("your Plan") if you are a Plan enrollee.

- You have the right to know about any decisions that the hospital, your doctor, your Plan, or anyone else makes about your hospital stay and who will pay for it.

- Your doctor, your Plan, or the hospital should arrange for services you will need after you leave the hospital. Medicare or your Plan may cover some care in your home (home health care) and other kinds of care, if ordered by your doctor or by your Plan. You have a right to know about these services, who will pay for them, and where you can get them. If you have any questions, talk to your doctor or Plan, or talk to other hospital personnel.

YOUR HOSPITAL DISCHARGE & MEDICARE APPEAL RIGHTS

Date of Discharge: When your doctor or Plan determines that you can be discharged from the hospital, you will be advised of your planned date of discharge. You may appeal if you think that you are being asked to leave the hospital too soon. If you stay in the hospital after your planned date of discharge, it is likely that your charges for additional days in the hospital will not be covered by Medicare or your Plan.

Your Right to an Immediate Appeal without Financial Risk: When you are advised of your planned date of discharge, if you think you are being asked to leave the hospital too soon, you have the right to appeal to your Quality Improvement Organization (also known as a QIO). The QIO is authorized by Medicare to provide a second opinion about your readiness to leave. You may call Medicare toll-free, 24 hours a day, at 1-800-MEDICARE (1-800-633-4227), or TTY/TTD: 1-877-486-2048, for more information on asking your QIO for a second opinion. If you appeal to the QIO by noon of the day after you receive a noncoverage notice, you are not responsible for paying for the days you stay in the hospital during the QIO review, even if the QIO disagrees with you. The QIO will decide within one day after it receives the necessary information.

Other Appeal Rights: If you miss the deadline for filing an immediate appeal, you may still request a review by the QIO (or by your Plan, if you are a Plan enrollee) before you leave the hospital. However, you will have to pay for the costs of your additional days in the hospital if the QIO (or your Plan) denies your appeal. You may file for this review at the address or telephone number of the QIO (or of your Plan).

OMB Approval No. 0938-0692.   Form No. CMS-R-193   (January 2003)

Figure 15-1 Printout Entitled "An Important Message from Medicare"

Both outpatient and emergency room procedures must be established so as to collect the maximum amount of information available at that time. Many admissions departments as well as emergency departments join online insurance verification systems so that payers can be contacted during the registration process and verification can be received in seconds.

Records of Treatments and Charges During the Hospital Stay

The patient's hospital medical record contains: (1) a face sheet (similar to a patient registration form that has been computer-generated); (2) notes of the attending physician, (and physician order sheets), and other treating physicians, such as operative reports; (3) ancillary documents like nurses' notes, medication administration records, and pathology, radiology, and laboratory reports; (4) patient data, including insurance information for patients who have been in the hospital before; and (5) a correspondence section that contains signed consent forms and other documents. In line with HIPAA security requirements, the confidentiality and security of patients' medical records are guarded by all hospital staff. Both technical means, such as passwords and encryption, and legal protections, such as requiring staff members to sign confidentiality pledges, are used to ensure privacy.

Inpatients are usually charged by hospitals for the following services (the *technical component* of procedures):

- Room and board
- Medications
- Ancillary tests and procedures, such as laboratory workups
- Equipment used during surgery or therapy
- The amount of time spent in an operating room, recovery room, or intensive care unit

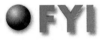

Physician's Fees
The professional fee for the physician's services, such as surgeon's fees, is charged by the physician rather than the hospital.

Patients are charged according to the type of accommodations and services they receive. For example, the rate for a private room is higher than for a semiprivate room, and intensive care unit or recovery room charges are higher than charges for standard rooms. When patients are transferred to these various services, this activity is tracked. In an outpatient or an emergency department encounter, there is no room and board charge; instead, there is a visit charge.

Average service charges vary according to the type of care the hospital provides. For example, at a one-hundred-bed hospital that provides basic services, a large bill may be $15,000; but at a large five-hundred-bed hospital performing complicated surgeries such as open-heart procedures, a large bill is often more than $100,000.

Discharge and Billing

Usually, by the time patients are discharged from the hospital, their accounts have been totaled and insurance claims or bills created. The goal in most cases is to file a claim or bill within seven days after discharge. The items are recorded on the hospital's charge description master file, usually called the charge master or charge ticket, which is similar to a medical office encounter form, but with many more entries. This master list contains the following information for each billable item:

- The hospital's code for the service and a brief description of it
- The charge for the service
- The hospital department (such as laboratory)
- The hospital's cost to provide the service
- A procedure code for the service

The hospital's computer system tracks the patient's services. For example, if the patient is sent to the intensive care unit after surgery, the intensive care department's billing group reports the specific items performed for the patient, and these charges are entered on the patient's account.

INPATIENT (HOSPITAL) CODING

The HIM department is also responsible for diagnostic and procedural coding of the patients' medical records. (based upon the discharge summary signed by the attending physician). Coding is done by inpatient medical coders as soon as the patient is discharged. Some inpatient coders are generalists; others may have special skills in a certain area, like surgical coding or Medicare. Volumes 1 and 2 of the ICD-9-CM are used to code inpatient diagnoses, and Volume 3 is used to code procedures performed during hospitalization.

Hospital Diagnostic Coding

Different rules apply for assigning inpatient codes than for those used for physician office diagnoses. The rules are extensive; three of them are described briefly below to illustrate some of the major differences in inpatient versus outpatient coding.

Rule 1—Principal Diagnosis

For ICD-9-CM diagnostic coding in medical practices, the first code listed is the primary diagnosis, defined as the main reason for the patient's encounter with the provider. Under hospital inpatient rules, the principal diagnosis is listed first. The principal diagnosis is the condition established *after study* to be chiefly responsible for this admission. This principal diagnosis is listed even if the patient has other, more severe diagnoses. In some cases, the admitting diagnosis—the condition identified by the physician at admission to the hospital—is also reported.

Rule 2—Suspected or Unconfirmed Diagnoses

When the patient is admitted for workups to uncover the cause of a problem, inpatient medical coders can also use a suspected or unconfirmed condition (rule out) if it is listed as the admitting diagnosis. The admitting diagnosis may not match the principal diagnosis once a final decision is made.

Rule 3—Comorbidities and Complications

The inpatient coder also lists all the other conditions that have an effect on the patient's hospital stay or course of treatment. A patient's other conditions at admission that affect care during the hospitalization are called comorbidities, meaning coexisting conditions. Conditions that develop as complications of surgery or other treatments are coded as complications.

Comorbidities and complications are shown in the patient medical record with the initials CC. Coding CCs is important because their presence may increase the hospital's reimbursement level for the care. The hospital insurance claim form discussed later in this chapter allows for up to eight additional conditions to be reported.

Hospital Procedural Coding

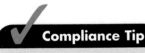

Compliance Tip

The inpatient coding rules apply only to inpatient services. Both hospital-based outpatient services and physician office services are reported using Volumes 1 and 2 of the ICD-9-CM, and using the outpatient rules and CPT codes for procedures.

In inpatient coding, ICD-9, Volume 3, Procedures, is used to assign procedure codes. Reporting Volume 3 codes when appropriately documented may increase the hospital's reimbursement level for a patient's care because some procedures require more hospital time for recovery. For example, codes in range 93.31 to 93.39 are assigned when patients require physical therapy procedures such as whirlpool therapy.

Volume 3 of the ICD-9-CM has an Alphabetic Index and a Tabular List similar to those in Volumes 1 and 2. The Alphabetic Index is used to locate the procedure, and the Tabular List is used to confirm the code selection. Codes are either three or four digits. The fourth digit must be assigned if available.

The principal procedure assigned by the inpatient medical coder is the procedure that is most closely related to the treatment of the principal diagnosis. It is usually a surgical procedure. If no surgery is performed, the principal procedure may be a therapeutic procedure.

PAYERS AND PAYMENT METHODS

Medicare and Medicaid both provide coverage for eligible patients' hospital services. Medicare Part A, known as hospital insurance, helps pay for inpatient hospital care, skilled nursing facilities (SNF), hospice care, and home health care. Private payers also offer hospitalization insurance. Most employees have coverage for hospital services through employers' programs.

Medicare Inpatient Payment System

Medicare's actions to control the cost of hospital services began with diagnosis-related groups (DRGs). Under the DRG classification system, the hospital stays of patients who had similar diagnoses were studied. Groupings were created based on the relative value of the resources that physicians and hospitals nationally used for patients with similar conditions. The calculations combine data about the patient's diagnosis and procedures with factors that affect the outcome of treatment, such as age, gender, comorbidities, and complications. At the same time the DRG system was created, Medicare changed the way hospitals were paid. Payment changed from a fee-for-service approach to the Medicare Prospective Payment System (PPS). In the PPS, the payment for each type of service is set ahead of time based on the DRG.

When DRGs were established, Medicare also set up Peer Review Organizations (PROs), which were later renamed Quality Improvement Organizations (QIOs). Made up of practicing physicians and other health care experts, these organizations are contracted by CMS in each state to review Medicare and Medicaid claims for the appropriateness of hospitalization and clinical care. QIOs aim to ensure that payment is made only for medically necessary services. QIOs are also resources for investigating patients' complaints regarding the quality of care at a given facility or through a managed care plan.

Medicare Outpatient Payment Systems

The use of DRGs under a PPS system proved to be very effective in controlling costs. In 2000 this approach was implemented for outpatient hospital services, which previously were paid on a fee-for-service basis. For example, the Hospital Outpatient Prospective Payment System (PPS) is used to pay for hospital outpatient services. In place of DRGs, patients are grouped under an ambulatory patient classification (APC) system. Reimbursement is made according to preset amounts based on the value of each APC.

Private Insurance Companies

Because of the expense involved with hospitalization, private payers encourage providers to minimize the number of days patients stay in the hospital. Most private payers establish the standard number of days allowed for various conditions and compare this number to the patient's actual stay. Many private payers have also adopted the DRG method of setting prospective payments for hospital services. Hospitals and the payers, which may include Blue Cross and Blue Shield or other managed care plans, negotiate the rates for each DRG.

CLAIMS AND FOLLOW UP

Hospitals must submit claims for Medicare Part A reimbursement to Medicare fiscal intermediaries using the HIPAA health care claim called 837I. Similar to the 837 claim (Chapter 6), this format is called I for "institutional"; the physicians' claim is called 837P for "professional."

In some situations, a paper claim form called the UB-92 (uniform billing 1992), also known as the CMS-1450, is also accepted by most other payers.

837I Health Care Claim Completion

The 837I, like the 837P, has sections requiring data elements for the billing and the pay-to provider, the subscriber and patient, and the payer, plus claim and service level details. Most of the data elements report the same information as summarized below for the paper claim.

UB-92 Claim Form Completion

The UB-92 claim form is complex; it has eighty-six data fields, some requiring multiple entries. The form is shown in Figure 15-2. It is used to report patient data, information on the insured, facility/patient type, the source of the admission, various conditions that affect payment, whether Medicare is

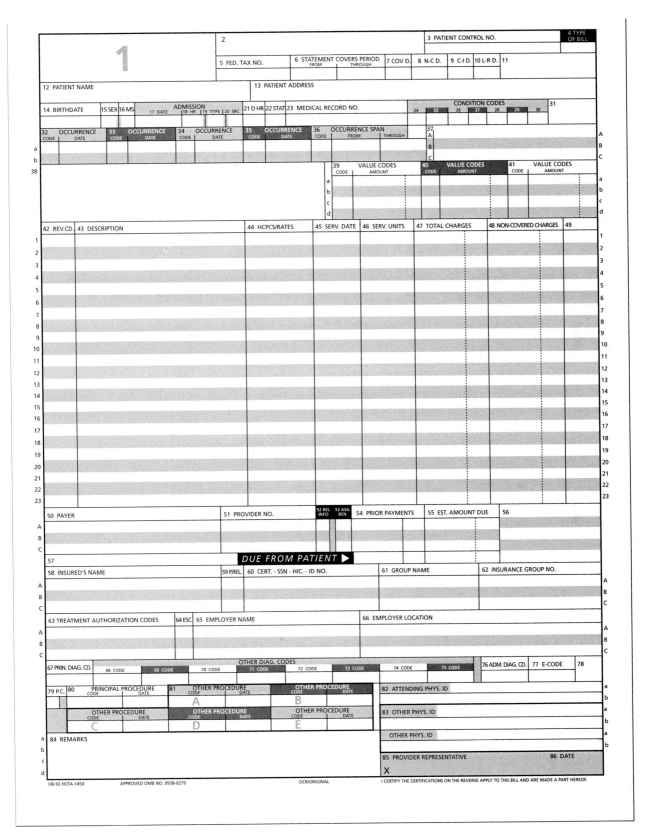

Figure 15–2 UB-92 Form

the primary payer (for Medicare claims), the principal and other diagnosis codes, the admitting diagnosis, the principal procedure code, the attending physician, other key physicians, and charges. The information for the form locators often requires choosing from a list of codes. All dates should show the year as four digits.

Remittance Advice Processing

Hospitals receive a remittance advice when payments are transmitted to their accounts. The patient accounting department and then the health information management (HIM) department check that appropriate payment has been received. Unless the software used for billing automatically reports if the billed code is not the same as the paid code, procedures to find and follow up these exceptions must be set up between the two departments.

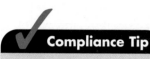

Compliance Tip

Like physician practice coding, the correct level of service must be reported to avoid fraud. For example, a patient has pulmonary edema (fluid in the lungs) that is due to the principal diagnosis of congestive heart failure (CHF). The correct ICD-9-CM code order leads to a DRG 127 classification. If the coder incorrectly reports pulmonary edema and respiratory failure, the patient is assigned DRG 87, which has a higher relative value, resulting in an improperly high payment.

Professional Focus

Career Opportunities in Hospitals

Provider Relations Representative

Provider relations representatives speak for an institution to its network of physicians. Because they establish networks of providers, many hospitals employ provider relations representatives to enroll physicians in their networks and to monitor their status. These employees process the documents needed for providers to become participants in the network, maintain the current list of providers, and answer questions from providers about policies and procedures.

Medical Coder—Hospital

Medical coding specialists who work in the hospital setting are called hospital or facility coders. They may work in an inpatient setting, an outpatient clinic, or another institution such as a skilled nursing facility. Hospital coders review patients' medical records and assign diagnosis and procedure codes. They are knowledgeable about the coding rules and procedures for hospital coding, and they may be certified by either the American Academy of Professional Coders (AAPC) or the American Health Information Management Association (AHIMA). Hospital coders need to become experienced in working with lengthy, complicated records of patients' stays, including operative, laboratory, pathology, and radiology reports. Accurate coding is a critical part of ensuring that claims follow the legal and ethical requirements of Medicare and other third-party payers.

Chapter Summary

1. Inpatient (involving an overnight stay) services are provided by general and specialized hospitals, skilled nursing facilities, and long-term care facilities. Outpatient services are provided by ambulatory surgical centers or units, by home health agencies, and by hospice staff.

2. The first major step in the hospital claims processing sequence is admission, when the patient is registered. Personal and financial information is entered in the hospital's health record system; insurance coverage is verified; and consent forms are signed by the patient. In the second step, the patient's treatments and transfer among the various departments in the hospital are tracked and recorded. The third step, discharge and billing, follows the discharge of the patient from the facility and completion of the patient's record. Payments are based upon the appropriate diagnosis-related group (DRG) and are set in advance (prospective in nature).

3. Two ways in which inpatient coding differs from physician and outpatient diagnostic coding are that (a) the main diagnosis, called the principal diagnosis, is established after study in the hospital setting, and (b) unconfirmed conditions (rule outs) may be coded as the admitting diagnosis.

4. Volume 3 of the ICD-9-CM, Procedures, is used to report the procedures for inpatient services. The three- or four-digit codes are assigned based on the principal diagnosis.

5. In hospital billing, the HIPAA claim for institutions, known as the 837I, or in some situations, the paper UB-92 claim form (CMS-1450), is used to report patient data, information on the insured, facility/patient type, the source of the admission, various conditions that affect payment, whether Medicare is the primary payer (for Medicare claims), the principal and other diagnosis codes, the admitting diagnosis, the principal procedure code, the attending physician, other key physicians, and charges.

Check Your Understanding

Part 1. **Write "T" or "F" in the blank to indicate whether you think the statement is true or false.**

_____ **1.** Skilled nursing facilities (SNF) are classified as outpatient facilities.

_____ **2.** Emergency care involves a life-threatening situation.

_____ **3.** An inpatient's insurance coverage is usually verified in the discharge process.

_____ **4.** The master patient index contains the name of each patient's attending physician.

_____ **5.** Hospital services are covered by Medicare Part A.

_____ **6.** At-home care is considered outpatient care.

_____ **7.** The hospital's charge master serves the same purpose as a medical office's encounter form.

_____ **8.** The principal diagnosis is based on the admitting diagnosis.

_____ **9.** Inpatient coding rules do not permit the reporting of suspected or unconfirmed diagnoses.

_____ **10.** ICD-9-CM, Volume 3, is used to report inpatient procedures.

Part 2. **Choose the best answer.**

_____ **1.** When the hospital staff collects data on a patient who is being admitted for services, the process is called:
   a. health information management
   b. registration
   c. MSP
   d. precertification

_____ **2.** Which of the following hospital departments has different procedures for collecting patients' personal and insurance information?
   a. accounting department
   b. surgery department
   c. emergency department
   d. collections department

_____ **3.** Patient charges in hospitals vary according to:
   a. their accommodations
   b. their services
   c. their accommodations and services
   d. their insurance coverage

_____ **4.** Conditions that arise during the patient's hospital stay as a result of treatments are called:
   a. comorbidities
   b. admitting diagnoses
   c. complications
   d. correlates

_____ **5.** In inpatient coding, the initials CC mean:
   a. chief complaint
   b. comorbidities and complications
   c. cubic centimeters
   d. convalescent center

_____ **6.** The code 76.23 is an example of which type of code?
   a. CPT-4
   b. ICD-9-CM, Volume 1
   c. ICD-9-CM, Volume 2
   d. ICD-9-CM, Volume 3

_____ **7.** Under a prospective payment system, payments for services are:
   a. set in advance
   b. calculated based on the provider's fees
   c. based on a discount to the provider's usual fees
   d. none of the above

_____ **8.** When preparing claims for Medicare Part A reimbursement, hospitals must use the:
   a. UB-92
   b. 837P
   c. CMS-1450
   d. 837I

Part 3. Why do the inpatient coding rules permit coding rule outs for diagnoses, and why do the physician office coding rules not allow them?

_____

_____

_____

_____

Chapter 16 first provides Part I, an introduction to the NDCMedisoft Advanced Patient Accounting program. Then, in Parts II and III, you will use the program to complete seven claims. In Part II you are given step-by-step instructions on completing Case Study 16-1 and optional Case Study 16-2. In Part III you will complete five claims on your own.

Part I Introduction to NDCMediSoft

The NDCMedisoft introduction is in two parts:

- An overview of NDCMedisoft is contained in a PDF file on the Student Data Disk located inside the back cover of this text. The PDF file (Overview-Medisoft.pdf) describes the program's database structure, how claims are created in NDCMedisoft, and the major dialog boxes that are used for data entry in creating claims.
- Getting Started with NDCMedisoft, which follows in the text below, contains hands-on instructions in getting started with the program, including setting up the NDCMedisoft database files that are used in the simulations in Parts II and III and practice in using NDCMedisoft menus.

Viewing the Overview on the PDF File

Note that the data you need are supplied on two media, a floppy disk and a CD-ROM. The instructions here assume the use of the Student Data Disk. If you are instead using the Student CD-ROM, ask your instructor for guidance in substituting these instructions with those specific to your computer's setup.

Before viewing the overview to NDCMedisoft on the Student Data Disk, follow the instructions below to make a working copy of the disk so that the original disk can be stored in a safe place. You may need the original disk to make another copy if the working copy is accidentally damaged or lost.

Making a Copy of the Student Data Disk

Note: These instructions assume that Windows 98 or a later version is installed on your computer.

1. Turn on the computer and monitor.
2. After the Windows desktop is displayed, insert the Student Data Disk in the A: drive. (If you are using a different drive, please substitute that letter for "A" whenever it appears.)
3. Locate the My Computer icon, either on the desktop or in the Start menu, and click it. The My Computer window is displayed.
4. In the My Computer window, click the icon labeled 3½ Floppy (A:).
5. Open the File menu, and select Copy Disk. The Copy Disk dialog box is displayed.
6. The Copy From and Copy To windows should both list 3½ Floppy (A:). If more than one item is listed in each window, click 3½ Floppy (A:) in both windows to select them.

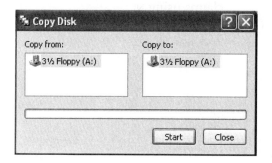

7. Click the Start button. (If a dialog box appears prompting you to insert the source disk, make sure the Student Data Disk is in the drive, and then click OK.)
8. The computer begins reading the files on the source disk. When the system prompts you to insert the disk you want to copy to (the destination disk), eject the Student Data Disk from the drive.
9. Insert a blank disk in the floppy drive, and click the OK button. The files are copied to the destination disk.
10. When the copy is completed, the message "Copy completed successfully" is displayed. Eject the disk from the drive, and label it "Working Copy CPC."
11. Close the Copy Disk dialog box.
12. Close the My Computer dialog box.

Now that you have a working copy of the Student Data Disk, follow these steps to view the overview:

To access Overview-Medisoft.pdf:

1. Turn on the computer and monitor.
2. After the Windows desktop is displayed, insert the working copy of the Student Data Disk in the 3½ floppy drive (drive A:).
3. Click the Start button on the Windows taskbar to display the Start menu.
4. Click the Run . . . option.
5. In the Run dialog box, key:

   a:Overview-Medisoft.pdf
6. Click the OK button. The file opens in Acrobat Reader. View the contents of the file for an introduction to the NDCMedisoft program.

Note: If you do not have the Acrobat Reader program on your system, ask your instructor or lab facilitator for help obtaining a copy.

Getting Started with NDCMedisoft

This section provides hands-on practice using NDCMedisoft for the first time with this text. You will start the program and restore the database files that are used in the claim simulations in Parts II and III. Then you will practice using NDCMedisoft menus.

As mentioned in the overview, before a medical office begins to create claims using NDCMedisoft, basic information about the practice must be entered in the computer. This preliminary work has been done for you and stored in a backup file on the Student Data Disk. The medical practice with which you will work is called Central Practice Center (CPC).

Starting NDCMedisoft and Restoring the Backup File

The following instructions take you through the steps of starting NDCMedisoft and restoring the backup file of the Central Practice Center database from the Student Data Disk onto the hard drive for future use. These steps only need to be followed once. You will create a new directory and data set name for the Central Practice Center files on the hard drive, and then restore the backup file to the new directory.

Thereafter, when the NDCMedisoft program is started, the required data set will load automatically, as the program is designed to open whatever database files it used during the previous session.

1. While holding down the F7 key, click Start, Programs, NDCMedisoft, and then NDCMedisoft Advanced Patient Accounting to start NDCMedisoft. When the Find NDCMedisoft Database dialog box appears, release the F7 key. This dialog box asks you to enter the NDCMedisoft data directory.

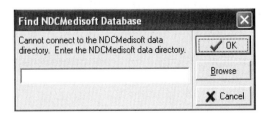

2. Click inside the data entry box to activate it. Then key *C:\MediData* in the space provided (where C is the letter that represents the hard drive you will be using). The dialog box should now look like this:

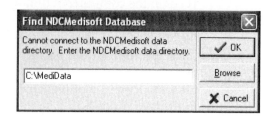

3. Click the OK button. An Information dialog box appears.

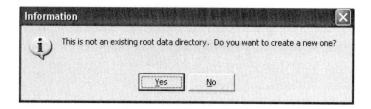

4. Click Yes. The Create Data dialog box is displayed.

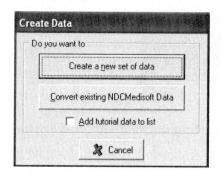

5. Click the Create a New Set of Data button. The Create a New Set of Data dialog box appears. In the upper box, key *Central Practice Center.* In the lower box, key *CPC.* The dialog box should now look like this:

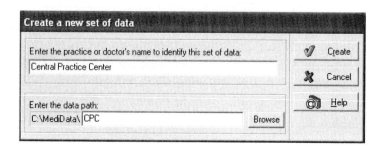

6. Click the Create button. A Confirm dialog box is displayed.

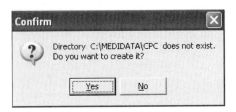

7. Click the Yes button. The Practice Information box appears. In the Practice Name box, key *Central Practice Center.* Leave the remaining boxes blank for now, as the backup file will fill them in later.

8. Click the Save button. The main window of the NDCMedisoft program is displayed, with the name of the new data set, Central Practice Center, on the title bar. Your screen should look like this:

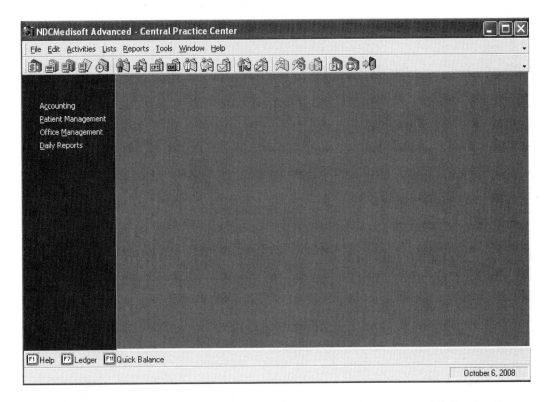

9. Insert the working copy of the Student Data Disk in the floppy drive. (If you are using a different drive, please substitute that letter for "A" whenever it appears.)

10. Open the File menu at the top of the window, and locate the Restore Data option halfway down the menu.

11. Click Restore Data. A Warning dialog box is displayed.

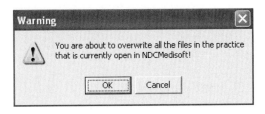

12. Click the OK button. The Restore dialog box is displayed. In the top box, key the filename *A:\CPC.mbk* if it does not already appear. This is the name of the file on the Student Data Disk. The dialog box should now look like this:

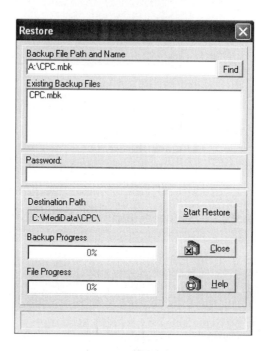

13. Click the Start Restore button. A Confirm dialog box is displayed.

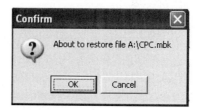

14. Click the OK button. After the program restores the database to the hard drive, an Information dialog box is displayed, indicating that the restore is complete. Click OK.
15. You are returned to the main NDCMedisoft window. (*Hint*: If the main NDCMedisoft window does not fill the screen, click the Maximize button to expand it.)
16. By default, NDCMedisoft displays a sidebar with four options on the left side of the window. As the sidebar is not required for this text, open the Window menu and click the Show Side Bar option to toggle it off.
17. The sidebar disappears. The database is now ready for use.
18. For now, keep the NDCMedisoft program open, as you will use the program when you practice using menus in the next section.

Practice Selecting Menu Options

NDCMedisoft offers program choices through a group of eight menus. The NDCMedisoft menu bar lists the name of each NDCMedisoft menu: File, Edit, Activities, Lists, Reports, Tools, Window, and Help. (A Services menu may also be available if the practice is sending electronic prescriptions.)

The two menus used the most in the NDCMedisoft exercises in this text are the Lists menu and the Activities menu.

The Lists Menu   Some of the data already entered for Central Practice Center is accessed through the Lists menu. Use the following steps to practice selecting some of the options on the Lists menu.

1. Click the menu name, Lists, to display the Lists menu.

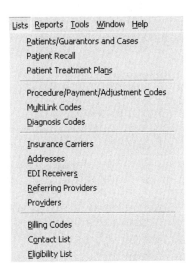

2. Click the first option, Patients/Guarantors and Cases. The Patient List dialog box is displayed. This dialog box contains the names and chart numbers of all the established patients for the medical office.
3. Click the Close button to return to the main NDCMedisoft window.
4. Again, click the menu name, Lists.
5. When the Lists menu is displayed, click Procedure/Payment/Adjustment Codes. The list that appears contains the CPT codes and descriptions for the procedures that are most frequently used by this medical office. Scroll to the bottom of the list. Notice the list also contains a number of codes for accounting purposes, such as take back, withhold, adjustment, copayment charge, copayment, deductible, and payment codes.
6. Click the Close button to return to the main NDCMedisoft window.

7. To learn more about the program, access two more options from the Lists menu, Diagnosis Codes and Insurance Carriers. The Diagnosis List dialog box lists the ICD codes and descriptions of the diagnoses that are most frequently used by this medical office. The Insurance Carrier List dialog box displays a list of the carriers where most of this office's claims are filed.

8. When you are finished viewing the lists, return to the main NDCMedisoft window.

The Activities Menu Other than the patients' personal and case information, much of the data necessary to create claims is entered through options on the Activities menu. Follow the steps below to view two major dialog boxes that are accessed through the Activities menu:

1. Click Activities on the menu bar to display the Activities menu.

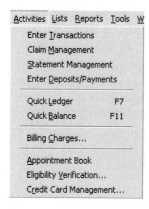

2. Click the first option, Enter Transactions. The Transaction Entry dialog box is displayed. This dialog box is used to enter data about patient transactions and to record charges and payments.

3. Click the Close button.

4. Again, open the Activities menu.

5. Click Claim Management. The dialog box that appears is used to create and transmit (or print) electronic and paper claims.

6. Click the Close button.

The menu options in NDCMedisoft provide insight into the type of data that is stored in the program. In Parts II and III, you will use the dialog boxes connected with these menus to create claims.

NOTE: Before completing the claim simulations in Part II, be sure you have followed the instructions in Part I, "Getting Started with NDCMedisoft," to restore the database files for Central Practice Center, the sample medical practice used in these simulations.

In Case Study 16-1 you will:
- Edit an established patient's record.
- Enter the patient's diagnosis code.
- Enter the transactions for an office visit.
- Print a walkout receipt.
- Create an electronic claim with a claim verification report.

Case Study 16-1

Robin Caruthers, an established patient at Central Practice Center, comes to the office for a routine visit. As the medical insurance specialist, you enter the transactions for the office visit. After entering the transactions, you create an electronic claim and view the claim verification report for the claim.

Follow the steps on pages 247–258 to complete Case Study 16-1.

Edit an Established Patient's Record

When Robin Caruthers arrives at the medical office for her routine appointment, you first ask her to verify her current address. You determine that her street address and phone number need to be updated. Follow these steps to correct Mrs. Caruthers' address:
1. Select Patients/Guarantors and Cases from the Lists menu.
2. When the Patient List dialog box appears, click Caruthers, Robin to highlight the entry.
3. Click the Edit Patient button in the bottom-left corner of the Patient List dialog box. The Patient/Guarantor dialog box for Robin Caruthers is displayed.
4. Press the Tab key three times to move to the Street field, or click in the Street box.
5. Key the correct street address, *22 Bayside Drive.*
6. Click in the Home (phone) box.
7. Edit the home phone to display *(602) 629-0222.* The Patient/Guarantor dialog box should look like the one on page 248.

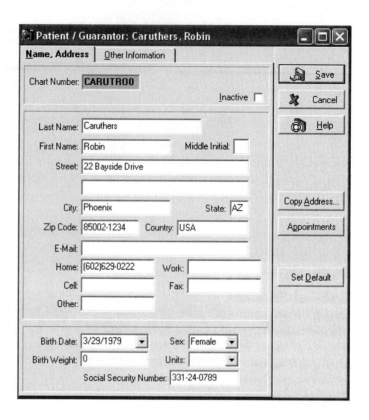

8. Click the Save button to save the changes and return to the Patient List dialog box.

....

Enter Diagnosis Information

After Mrs. Caruthers finishes her appointment with the doctor, she hands you the encounter form from the visit. Before you can enter the transactions on the encounter form, you need to enter the diagnosis code on the encounter form in Mrs. Caruthers' Case dialog box. In NDCMedisoft, transactions must be linked to at least one diagnosis code. If they are not, the claim created for the transactions will be rejected by the insurance company.

1. With Robin Caruthers' Chart Number and Case information still displayed in the Patient List dialog box, click the line that reads Ventricular Fibrillation on the right side of the dialog box to select this case.
2. Click the Edit Case button at the bottom of the dialog box.
3. The nine tabs for this case appear. Click the Diagnosis tab.
4. Notice that the four Default Diagnosis boxes are blank. As today's appointment was a routine visit in connection with her ventricular fibrillation case, the diagnosis code on the encounter form is 427.41 (Ventricular Fibrillation). In the Default Diagnosis 1 box, key the first two numbers of this code to highlight the diagnosis code for Ventricular Fibrillation.

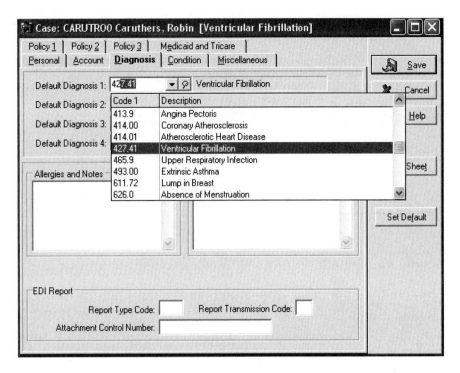

5. Press Enter to select the diagnosis, and then click the Save button to save your work.
6. Click the Close button to exit the Patient List dialog box.

Enter New Transactions

Now that Robin Caruthers' diagnosis code has been recorded, follow the steps below to enter the transactions for the visit. In addition to the encounter form, Mrs. Caruthers hands you a check for $20 because her PPO requires a $20 copay per visit. Therefore, there are three transactions to be recorded for Mrs. Caruthers' visit today—a procedural charge for the office visit, a copayment charge, and a copayment.

1. Select Enter Transactions from the Activities menu to display the Transaction Entry dialog box.
2. Key *C* in the Chart box to locate the entry for Robin Caruthers, and then press Enter to display her information.

3. Notice that Robin Caruthers' current case (Ventricular Fibrillation) and insurance information, including her policy copayment requirement, are displayed in the top section of the Transaction Entry dialog box.

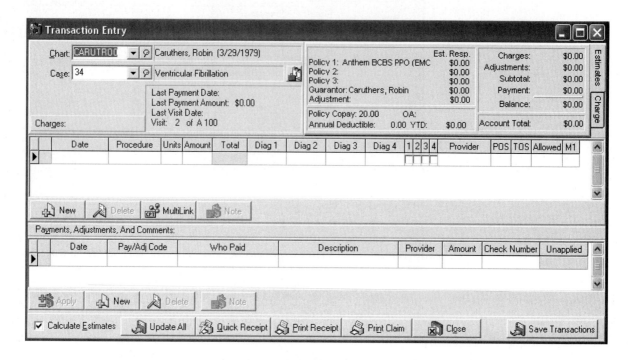

4. To enter a charge transaction, click the New button in the middle of the Transaction Entry dialog box, in the section labeled Charges.
5. Today's date is displayed as the default date in the Date field. Change the date in the Date box to 10/16/2008 by clicking inside the Date box and then keying *10162008* over the current entry.
6. Press the Tab key to move to the Procedure field.
7. Click the Triangle button in the Procedure field. A drop-down list of procedure codes and descriptions is displayed.
8. From Mrs. Caruthers' encounter form, you see that the procedure code for today's visit is 99212 (EP Problem focused). First key *9* in the Procedure box. Notice that the first code beginning with 9 is highlighted.
9. Key another *9*, and then key the rest of the procedure code—*212*—and press the Tab key. NDCMedisoft inserts the code in the Procedure box and displays the default unit of 1 in the Units box and the default amount of $46.00 in the Amount box. Notice that the Diagnosis code entered earlier in the Case dialog box, 427.41, is also displayed.

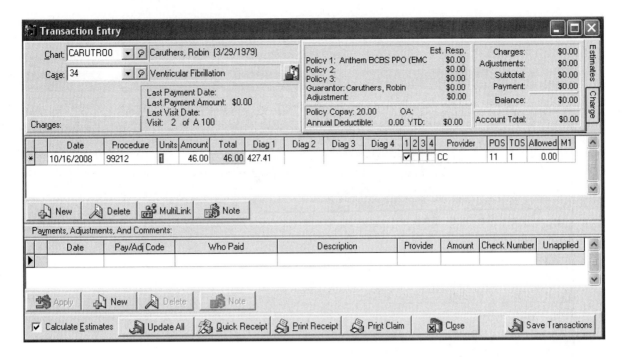

10. As Mrs. Caruthers' policy requires a $20 copay per visit, click the New button again to enter a second charge transaction for the copayment charge. (An Information box is displayed to remind you that Robin Caruthers' insurance requires a $20.00 copayment for each visit. Click the OK button to continue.)

11. Click the New button again. Make sure the date in the Date box is 10/16/2008. Press the Tab key to move to the Procedure box.

12. Click the Triangle button to display the list of codes.

13. Scroll to the bottom of the list to locate the code for Mrs. Caruthers' copayment charge. (Notice, at the top of the Transaction Entry dialog box, that her insurance carrier is Anthem BCBS PPO. Therefore, you are looking for the copayment charge for this carrier.) Click the code ANPCOPAY for "Anthem BCBS PPO Copayment Charge" to insert it in the Procedure box, and then press the Tab key.

14. NDCMedisoft displays the default amount of $20.00 in the Amount box.

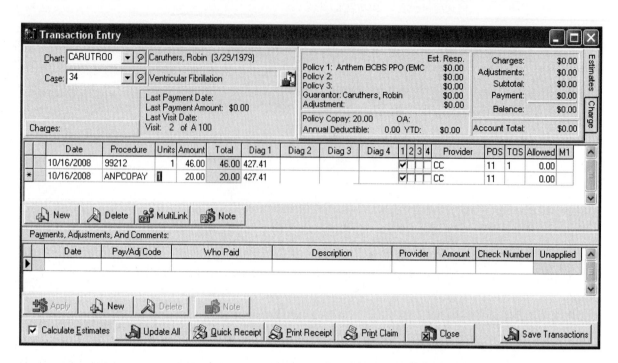

15. Now you will enter Mrs. Caruthers' payment. Payments are entered in the bottom section of the Transaction Entry dialog box. Click the New button in the Payments, Adjustments, and Comments section at the bottom of the dialog box.
16. Make sure the date in the Date field is still 10/16/2008. Then press the Tab key to move to the Pay/Adj Code box.
17. Click the Triangle button in this box to display the list of payment codes and descriptions. Scroll through the list to locate the "Anthem BCBS PPO Copayment" (ANPCPAY) code. Click the code, and then press Tab.
18. NDCMedisoft inserts the code in the Pay/Adj Code box and displays the name of the guarantor in the Who Paid box, and the default amount of "-20.00" in the Amount box for this transaction. The minus sign indicates a payment rather than a charge. Notice the Unapplied box at the end of the transaction line also displays the amount of the payment.

19. Click inside the Check Number box, and then key 339 to record the number on Mrs. Caruthers' check. The dialog box should now look like this:

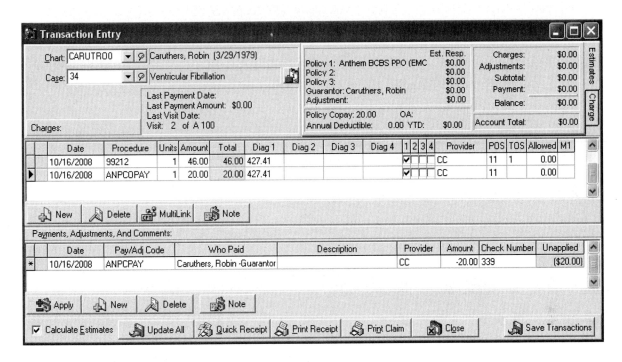

20. The last step in recording the payment is to apply the payment just entered to its corresponding charge. To do this, click the Apply button in the Payments, Adjustments, and Comments section of the dialog box.

21. The Apply Payment to Charges dialog box appears. Click the white background of the This Payment box on the line that contains the $20.00 copayment charge (line 2). The box is then outlined with a dashed line.

22. Key *20* and press Enter. The payment appears in the This Payment column. The copayment has now been applied to the corresponding copayment charge.

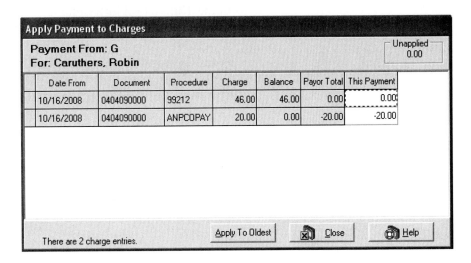

23. Click the Close button to close the Apply Payment to Charges dialog box.
24. Notice the amount in the Unapplied box at the end of the transaction line is now $0.00. Click the Save Transactions button in the lower right corner of the Transaction Entry dialog box to save the information you have entered in the Transaction Entry dialog box.
25. If the date of the transactions you are saving (10/16/2008) is later than the current date on your computer system, NDCMedisoft will display a Date of Service Validation box for each new transaction before it saves the transaction. This box asks you to confirm that you want to save the transaction, even though it has a future date.

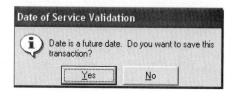

26. For the purposes of the simulations in this book, click Yes each time this box appears. In the present Transaction Entry screen, you will need to click Yes three times, as there are three new transactions.

You have successfully recorded two charges and one payment in the Transaction Entry dialog box. You can keep the Transaction Entry dialog box with Robin Caruthers' transactions open, as you will use it in the next section.

Create a Walkout Receipt

If a patient makes a payment during an office visit, the patient is usually given a walkout receipt at the time of the visit. After the transactions for the visit have been entered in the Transaction Entry dialog box, the Print Receipt button at the bottom of the Transaction Entry dialog box is used to print a walkout receipt. Follow these steps to create a walkout receipt for Robin Caruthers' visit.

1. With Robin Caruthers' transactions for 10/16/2008 still displayed in the Transaction Entry dialog box, click the Print Receipt button. (*Note*: Although the Quick Receipt button can also be used to print a walkout receipt, because of the likely difference in your computer's system date and the date used in the simulations, the Print Receipt button should be used in these simulations.)
2. The Open Report dialog box appears. The option Walkout Receipt (All Transactions) should be highlighted. If it is not, click this option to highlight it, and then click the OK button.
3. The Print Report Where? Dialog box appears, giving you the option to print the report, view it on screen, or export it to a file. If you are connected to a printer, select the Print the Report on the Printer option. (If you do not have a printer available, select the Preview the Report on the Screen option.) Then click the Start button.

4. The Walkout Receipt (All Transactions): Data Selections Questions dialog box appears. In both the Date From Range boxes in this dialog box, key *10162008* to change the date to 10/16/2008.

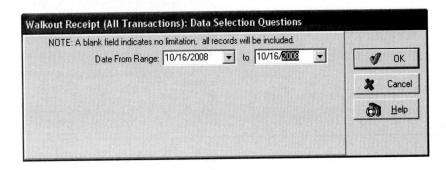

5. With the date range specified, click the OK button.
6. When the Print dialog box appears, click the OK button to begin printing. (If you chose to preview the report on screen, this box will not appear.)
7. After a few seconds, the receipt will be printed. (If you are previewing the walkout receipt on screen, it will appear in a Print Preview window. Click the Close button at the top of the screen when you are finished viewing it to exit the Print Preview window.)
8. After printing or viewing the walkout receipt, you are back at the Transaction Entry dialog box. Click the Close button to close the Transaction Entry dialog box.

Create an Electronic Claim and Print a Claim Verification Report

In most medical offices, claims are created and transmitted in batches, often at the end of the day. The batch method is more efficient, given the number of claims that are created daily. For instructional purposes, in this book claims are created and viewed as soon as the transactions for the claim have been recorded. The method of creating and sending claims is the same in both cases. When individual claims are created, the filtering option is set to a single chart number. When more than one claim is created, a range of chart numbers is specified. Follow the steps below to create an electronic claim for Robin Caruthers' transactions on 10/16/08.

Note: Because you are in an instructional setting and your system is not set up to send claims, you will not actually be able to transmit the claim electronically. This is the case for all the electronic claims in the simulations in this chapter. However, you will go through the steps leading up to the point of transmission, including verifying the details of the claim in a claim verification report.

1. To create a claim, click Claim Management on the Activities menu. The Claim Management dialog box is displayed. Claims that have already been created are listed in the dialog box.
2. To create a new claim, click the Create Claims button. The Create Claims dialog box appears. This dialog box is used to set the range of claims you want to create. In this instance, to enter the date 10/16/2008, key *10162008* in both of the Transaction Dates range boxes. (You may also change the date by clicking the triangle button to display a calendar, and then setting the appropriate date on the calendar.)

3. Depending on your computer's system date, when you enter the 10/16/2008 date, the program may display a Confirm box, asking if you want to change the future date you have entered. In both instances, click No and continue.

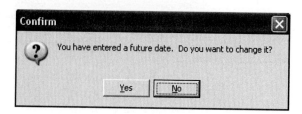

4. In both of the Chart Numbers range boxes, to select the claim for Robin Caruthers, key *C* and then press Enter. Leave the other boxes blank. (*Note:* If you were creating claims for all the patients' transactions during the day, you would enter today's date in the Transaction Dates boxes and leave the Chart Numbers boxes blank to select all chart numbers.)

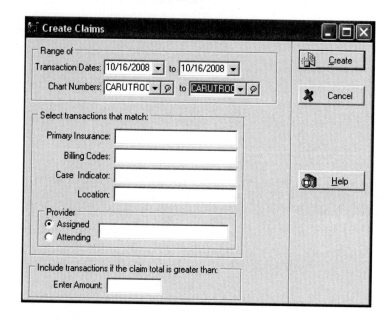

5. To create the claim for the transactions indicated, click the Create button.
6. The Create Claim dialog box closes, and you are returned to the Claim Management dialog box. Notice that the claim for Robin Caruthers is added to the list of created claims in the Claim Management dialog box. The Status 1 column in the Claim Management dialog box indicates the claim is "Ready to Send," and the Media 1 column indicates that the claim will be sent as an electronic file (EDI, "electronic data interchange"). This is because the default claim type for Mrs. Caruthers' insurance carrier is set to electronic.
7. To send the claim for Robin Caruthers to the clearinghouse, first make sure her claim is still selected in the Claim Management dialog box, and then click the Print/Send button.

8. The Print/Send Claims dialog box appears. Because Robin Caruthers' claim is an electronic claim, click the Electronic radio button in the billing method portion of the dialog box. In the Electronic Claim Receiver box, select NDC, which stands for National Data Corporation, the name of the clearinghouse, if it is not already selected.

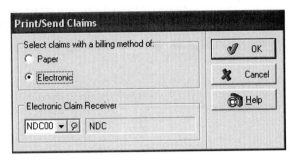

9. Click the OK button.
10. The Send Electronic Claims dialog box is displayed, with NDC displayed as the receiver. Click the Send Claims Now button.

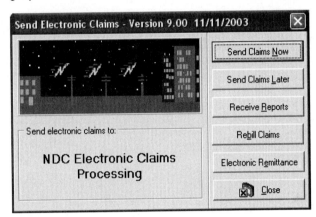

11. The Data Selection Questions dialog box appears. The various range boxes provide options for filtering the claims. In the first Chart Number Range box, key C to select Robin Caruthers, and then press Enter. Follow the same steps to fill in the second Chart Number Range box.

12. For the purposes of this simulation, delete the date displayed in the second Date Created Range box.

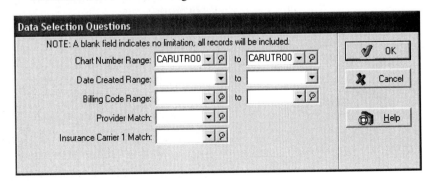

13. Click the OK button.

14. An Information dialog box appears, asking if you want to view a Verification report. Click the Yes button.
15. The Preview Report window appears with a copy of an EMC Verification report displayed. The report contains all the details of Robin Caruthers' claim, which is the only claim in the batch.

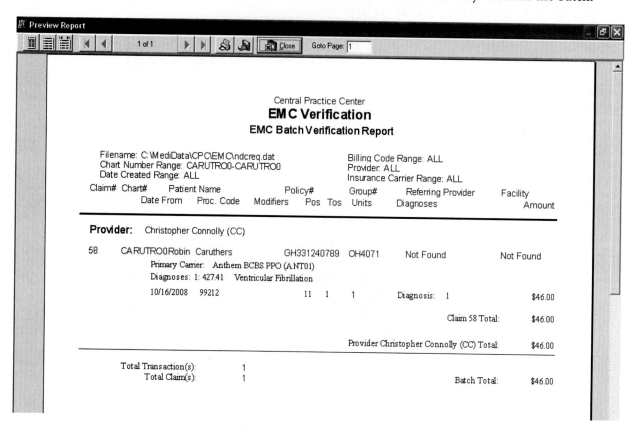

16. Click the Close button when finished viewing the report. The Preview Report window closes, and an Information dialog box appears, asking you if you want to continue with the transmission.

17. If you were in a medical office, you would click the Yes button and the claim would be sent electronically (for example, over a high-speed cable line) from your computer to a computer at the clearinghouse. However, because you are in a school setting and are not actually set up to submit electronic claims at this time, click the No button.
18. The Information dialog box disappears and the Claim Management dialog box appears as before. Because Robin Caruthers' claim was not actually sent, the "Ready to Send" status still appears. If the claim had actually been sent electronically, the Status 1 column would now read "Sent."
19. Click the Close button to close the Claim Management dialog box and return to the main NDCMedisoft window.

You have successfully completed Case Study 16-1.

Case Study 16-2

Additional guided practice in using NDCMedisoft to create claims is available by printing out Case Study 16-2, located on a PDF file on the Student Data Disk (CaseStudy16-2.pdf).

Similar to Case Study 16-1, Case Study 16-2 provides step-by-step instructions.

In Case Study 16-2 you will:

- Enter insurance information for a new patient.
- Enter the patient's diagnosis code.
- Enter the transactions for an office visit.
- Create and print a paper claim.

To access CaseStudy16-2.pdf:
1. Turn on the computer and monitor.
2. After the Windows desktop is displayed, insert the working copy of the Student Data Disk in the 3½ floppy drive (drive A:).
3. Click the Start button on the Windows taskbar to display the Start menu.
4. Click the Run . . . option.
5. In the Run dialog box, key:
    a:CaseStudy16-2.pdf
6. Click the OK button. The file opens in Acrobat Reader.
7. Print out the file, and then follow the steps to create a workers' compensation claim for Shih-Chi Yang, using NDCMedisoft.

Note: If you do not have the Acrobat Reader program on your system, ask your instructor or lab facilitator for help obtaining a copy.

Backing Up Data While Exiting NDCMedisoft

When entering data in NDCMedisoft, it is important to back up your work regularly for safekeeping. A backup copy of the database files prevents you from losing your work if the hard drive fails, or if you accidentally delete data while working. If you are working in an instructional environment where you share computers, it is essential that you back up your work on exiting the program, so that you can restore it at the beginning of the next session.

In the next section, you will back up the data entered during the last two simulations.

1. You can back up your data at any time using the Backup option on the File menu. However, by default, NDCMedisoft also gives you the opportunity to back up your data each time you exit the program. Click the Exit option on the File menu to exit NDCMedisoft.

2. The Backup Reminder dialog box appears. You will back up your data to your working copy of the Student Data Disk. First, make sure your working copy is in drive A:. Then click the Back Up Data Now button.

3. The Backup dialog box appears. The Destination File Path and Name box at the top should already read A:\CPC.mbk. If it does not, edit the top box so that it looks like the following, and then click the Start Backup button:

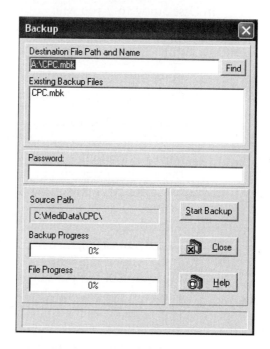

4. A Warning box displays the following message, "Backup file already exists. Do you want to replace it?" Click Yes.

5. NDCMedisoft backs up the data to the backup file in drive A:, and then displays an Information box indicating that the backup is complete.

6. Click the OK button to close the Information dialog box and exit the NDCMedisoft program.

Restoring a Backup File

If you are sharing a computer with other students in an instructional environment, you will need to perform a restore before a new NDCMedisoft session to be certain you are working with your own data. If necessary, follow these steps to restore your latest backup file:

To restore A:\CPC.mbk to C:\MediData\CPC:

1. Start NDCMedisoft.

2. Check the program's title bar at the top of the screen to make sure the Central Practice Center data set is the active data set. (If it is not, use the Open Practice option on the File menu to select it.)
3. Insert your working copy of the Student Data Disk in Drive A:.
4. Open the File menu and click Restore Data.
5. When the Warning box appears, click OK.
6. The Restore dialog box appears.

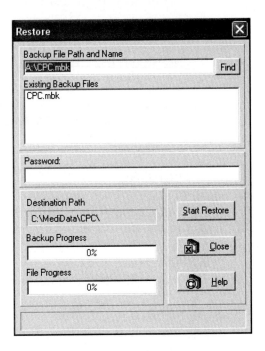

7. In the Backup File Path and Name box at the top of the dialog box, the following filename should already be displayed, *A:\CPC.mbk*. (If it is not, key it now.)
8. The Destination Path at the bottom of the box should already say C:\MediData\CPC. Leave this as it is.
9. Click the Start Restore button.
10. When the Confirm box appears, click OK.
11. An Information dialog box appears indicating the restore is complete. Click OK to continue.
12. The Restore dialog box disappears. You are ready to begin the next session.

In Part III, you will complete five claim simulations on your own, using what you learned in the guided simulations in Part II. Each simulation will test your knowledge of a different type of medical insurance:

- Case Study 16-3   Blue Cross and Blue Shield (PPO)
- Case Study 16-4   Medicare
- Case Study 16-5   Medicaid (HMO)
- Case Study 16-6   TRICARE
- Case Study 16-7   Workers' Compensation

For each of the five case studies, the following information has already been entered in the database from the patient information form: provider information, patient information, and insurance coverage. You will use the encounter form provided in each case study to carry out the remaining tasks:

1. Enter a diagnosis code.
2. Enter office visit transactions.
3. Print a walkout receipt (if a payment is received from the patient).
4. Create an electronic claim with a claim verification report.

If, during these simulations, you have questions about any procedures, notify your instructor or lab facilitator.

REMINDER: If you are in an instructional environment where you share computers, you may need to restore your work from the previous session before you begin the simulations in Part III of this chapter. See the instructions on Restoring a Backup File above (pp. 260–261).

CENTRAL PRACTICE CENTER
Vijay Singh, M.D.–Cardiovascular Disease
1122 E. University Drive
Mesa, AZ 85204
602–969–4237

PATIENT NAME	APPT. DATE/TIME
John O'Rourke	10/20/2006　　11:00am

PATIENT NO.	DX
OROURJO0	**1.** 414.00 coronary artherosclerosis

PAYMENT RECEIVED	**2.**
	3.
$20 copay, check #1922	**4.**

DESCRIPTION	✓	CPT	FEE	DESCRIPTION	✓	CPT	FEE
EXAMINATION				**PROCEDURES**			
New Patient				Diagnostic Anoscopy		46600	
Problem Focused		99201		ECG Complete	✓	93000	70
Expanded Problem Focused		99202		I&D, Abscess		10060	
Detailed	✓	99203	103	Pap Smear		88150	
Comprehensive		99204		Removal of Cerumen		69210	
Comprehensive/Complex		99205		Removal 1 Lesion		17000	
Established Patient				Removal 2-14 Lesions		17003	
Minimum		99211		Removal 15+ Lesions		17004	
Problem Focused		99212		Rhythm ECG w/Report		93040	
Expanded Problem Focused		99213		Rhythm ECG w/Tracing		93041	
Detailed		99214		Sigmoidoscopy, diag.		45330	
Comprehensive/Complex		99215					
				LABORATORY			
				Bacteria Culture		87081	
PREVENTIVE VISIT				Fungal Culture		87101	
New Patient				Glucose Finger Stick		82948	
Age 12-17		99384		Lipid Panel	✓	80061	64
Age 18-39		99385		Specimen Handling		99000	
Age 40-64		99386		Stool/Occult Blood		82270	
Age 65+		99387		Tine Test		85008	
Established Patient				Tuberculin PPD		85590	
Age 12-17		99394		Urinalysis		81000	
Age 18-39		99395		Venipuncture	✓	36415	16
Age 40-64		99396					
Age 65+		99397		**INJECTION/IMMUN.**			
				DT Immun		90702	
CONSULTATION: OFFICE/ER				Hepatitis A Immun		90632	
Requested By:				Hepatitis B Immun		90746	
Problem Focused		99241		Influenza Immun		90659	
Expanded Problem Focused		99242		Pneumovax		90732	
Detailed		99243					
Comprehensive		99244					
Comprehensive/Complex		99245		**TOTAL FEES**			

CENTRAL PRACTICE CENTER

Christopher Connolly, M.D.–General Practice
1122 E. University Drive
Mesa, AZ 85204
602–969–4237

PATIENT NAME	APPT. DATE/TIME
Donna Gaeta	10/07/2008 3:30pm

PATIENT NO.	DX
GAETADO0	**1.** v70.0 routine medical exam
PAYMENT RECEIVED	**2.**
	3.
	4.

DESCRIPTION	✓	CPT	FEE	DESCRIPTION	✓	CPT	FEE
EXAMINATION				**PROCEDURES**			
New Patient				Diagnostic Anoscopy		46600	
Problem Focused		99201		ECG Complete	✓	93000	29
Expanded Problem Focused		99202		I&D, Abscess		10060	
Detailed		99203		Pap Smear	✓	88150	29
Comprehensive		99204		Removal of Cerumen		69210	
Comprehensive/Complex		99205		Removal 1 Lesion		17000	
Established Patient				Removal 2-14 Lesions		17003	
Minimum		99211		Removal 15+ Lesions		17004	
Problem Focused		99212		Rhythm ECG w/Report		93040	
Expanded Problem Focused		99213		Rhythm ECG w/Tracing		93041	
Detailed		99214		Sigmoidoscopy, diag.		45330	
Comprehensive/Complex		99215					
				LABORATORY			
PREVENTIVE VISIT				Bacteria Culture		87081	
New Patient				Fungal Culture		87101	
Age 12-17		99384		Glucose Finger Stick		82948	
Age 18-39		99385		Lipid Panel		80061	
Age 40-64		99386		Specimen Handling		99000	
Age 65+	✓	99387	142	Stool/Occult Blood		82270	
Established Patient				Tine Test		85008	
Age 12-17		99394		Tuberculin PPD		85590	
Age 18-39		99395		Urinalysis	✓	81000	16
Age 40-64		99396		Venipuncture	✓	36415	16
Age 65+		99397					
				INJECTION/IMMUN.			
CONSULTATION: OFFICE/ER				DT Immun		90702	
Requested By:				Hepatitis A Immun		90632	
Problem Focused		99241		Hepatitis B Immun		90746	
Expanded Problem Focused		99242		Influenza Immun		90659	
Detailed		99243		Pneumovax		90732	
Comprehensive		99244					
Comprehensive/Complex		99245					
				TOTAL FEES			

CENTRAL PRACTICE CENTER
David Rosenberg, M.D.–Dermatology
1122 E. University Drive
Mesa, AZ 85204
602–969–4237

PATIENT NAME	APPT. DATE/TIME
Otto Kaar	10/14/2008 1:30pm

PATIENT NO.	DX
KAAROTT0	1. 682.1 abscess on neck

PAYMENT RECEIVED	2. 3.
$15 copay, check #331	4.

DESCRIPTION	✓	CPT	FEE	DESCRIPTION	✓	CPT	FEE
EXAMINATION				**PROCEDURES**			
New Patient				Diagnostic Anoscopy		46600	
Problem Focused		99201		ECG Complete		93000	
Expanded Problem Focused		99202		I&D, Abscess	✓	10060	57
Detailed		99203		Pap Smear		88150	
Comprehensive		99204		Removal of Cerumen		69210	
Comprehensive/Complex		99205		Removal 1 Lesion		17000	
Established Patient				Removal 2-14 Lesions		17003	
Minimum		99211		Removal 15+ Lesions		17004	
Problem Focused		99212		Rhythm ECG w/Report		93040	
Expanded Problem Focused	✓	99213	39	Rhythm ECG w/Tracing		93041	
Detailed		99214		Sigmoidoscopy, diag.		45330	
Comprehensive/Complex		99215					
				LABORATORY			
PREVENTIVE VISIT				Bacteria Culture		87081	
New Patient				Fungal Culture		87101	
Age 12-17		99384		Glucose Finger Stick		82948	
Age 18-39		99385		Lipid Panel		80061	
Age 40-64		99386		Specimen Handling		99000	
Age 65+		99387		Stool/Occult Blood		82270	
Established Patient				Tine Test		85008	
Age 12-17		99394		Tuberculin PPD		85590	
Age 18-39		99395		Urinalysis		81000	
Age 40-64		99396		Venipuncture		36415	
Age 65+		99397					
				INJECTION/IMMUN.			
CONSULTATION: OFFICE/ER				DT Immun		90702	
Requested By:				Hepatitis A Immun		90632	
Problem Focused		99241		Hepatitis B Immun		90746	
Expanded Problem Focused		99242		Influenza Immun		90659	
Detailed		99243		Pneumovax		90732	
Comprehensive		99244					
Comprehensive/Complex		99245		**TOTAL FEES**			

CENTRAL PRACTICE CENTER

Nancy Ronkowski, M.D.–Obstetrics & Gynecology
1122 E. University Drive
Mesa, AZ 85204
602–969–4237

PATIENT NAME				APPT. DATE/TIME			
Robyn Janssen				10/13/2008 10:00am			

PATIENT NO.				DX			
JANSSRO0				**1.** 626.0 absence of menstruation			

PAYMENT RECEIVED				**2.**			
$10 copay, check #2088				**3.** **4.**			

DESCRIPTION	✓	CPT	FEE	DESCRIPTION	✓	CPT	FEE
EXAMINATION				**PROCEDURES**			
New Patient				Diagnostic Anoscopy		46600	
Problem Focused		99201		ECG Complete		93000	
Expanded Problem Focused		99202		I&D, Abscess		10060	
Detailed		99203		Pap Smear		88150	
Comprehensive		99204		Removal of Cerumen		69210	
Comprehensive/Complex		99205		Removal 1 Lesion		17000	
Established Patient				Removal 2-14 Lesions		17003	
Minimum		99211		Removal 15+ Lesions		17004	
Problem Focused		99212		Rhythm ECG w/Report		93040	
Expanded Problem Focused	✓	99213	62	Rhythm ECG w/Tracing		93041	
Detailed		99214		Sigmoidoscopy, diag.		45330	
Comprehensive/Complex		99215					
				LABORATORY			
PREVENTIVE VISIT				Bacteria Culture		87081	
New Patient				Fungal Culture		87101	
Age 12-17		99384		Glucose Finger Stick		82948	
Age 18-39		99385		Lipid Panel		80061	
Age 40-64		99386		Specimen Handling		99000	
Age 65+		99387		Stool/Occult Blood		82270	
Established Patient				Tine Test		85008	
Age 12-17		99394		Tuberculin PPD		85590	
Age 18-39		99395		Urinalysis		81000	
Age 40-64		99396		Venipuncture		36415	
Age 65+		99397					
				INJECTION/IMMUN.			
CONSULTATION: OFFICE/ER				DT Immun		90702	
Requested By:				Hepatitis A Immun		90632	
Problem Focused		99241		Hepatitis B Immun		90746	
Expanded Problem Focused		99242		Influenza Immun		90659	
Detailed		99243		Pneumovax		90732	
Comprehensive		99244					
Comprehensive/Complex		99245					
				TOTAL FEES			

CENTRAL PRACTICE CENTER

Christopher Connolly, M.D.–General Practice
1122 E. University Drive
Mesa, AZ 85204
602–969–4237

PATIENT NAME	APPT. DATE/TIME
Marilyn Grogan	10/16/2008　　10:30am

PATIENT NO.	DX
GROGAMA0	**1.** 465.9 upper respiratory infection
PAYMENT RECEIVED	**2.**
	3.
	4.

DESCRIPTION	✓	CPT	FEE	DESCRIPTION	✓	CPT	FEE
EXAMINATION				**PROCEDURES**			
New Patient				Diagnostic Anoscopy		46600	
Problem Focused	✓	99201	56	ECG Complete		93000	
Expanded Problem Focused		99202		I&D, Abscess		10060	
Detailed		99203		Pap Smear		88150	
Comprehensive		99204		Removal of Cerumen		69210	
Comprehensive/Complex		99205		Removal 1 Lesion		17000	
Established Patient				Removal 2-14 Lesions		17003	
Minimum		99211		Removal 15+ Lesions		17004	
Problem Focused		99212		Rhythm ECG w/Report		93040	
Expanded Problem Focused		99213		Rhythm ECG w/Tracing		93041	
Detailed		99214		Sigmoidoscopy, diag.		45330	
Comprehensive/Complex		99215					
				LABORATORY			
PREVENTIVE VISIT				Bacteria Culture		87081	
New Patient				Fungal Culture	✓	87101	35
Age 12-17		99384		Glucose Finger Stick		82948	
Age 18-39		99385		Lipid Panel		80061	
Age 40-64		99386		Specimen Handling		99000	
Age 65+		99387		Stool/Occult Blood		82270	
Established Patient				Tine Test		85008	
Age 12-17		99394		Tuberculin PPD		85590	
Age 18-39		99395		Urinalysis		81000	
Age 40-64		99396		Venipuncture		36415	
Age 65+		99397					
				INJECTION/IMMUN.			
CONSULTATION: OFFICE/ER				DT Immun		90702	
Requested By:				Hepatitis A Immun		90632	
Problem Focused		99241		Hepatitis B Immun		90746	
Expanded Problem Focused		99242		Influenza Immun		90659	
Detailed		99243		Pneumovax		90732	
Comprehensive		99244					
Comprehensive/Complex		99245					
				TOTAL FEES			

Glossary

837I The HIPAA (ASC X12N) institutional claim transaction.

837P (HIPAA 837 claim) The HIPAA (ASC X12N) professional claim transaction.

A

acceptance of assignment (V. accept assignment) A participating physician's agreement to accept the allowed charge as payment in full.

accounts receivable (A/R) Monies owed to a medical practice by its patients and third-party payers.

Acknowledgment of Receipt of Notice of Privacy Practices Form accompanying a covered entity's Notice of Privacy Practices; covered entities must make a good-faith effort to have patients sign the acknowledgment.

acute Describes an illness or condition having severe symptoms and a short duration; can also refer to a sudden exacerbation of a chronic condition.

ADA Dental Claim Form Authorized form for submitting dental insurance claims.

add-on code Procedures that are performed and reported only in addition to a primary procedure; indicated in CPT by a plus sign (+) next to the code.

adjudication The process followed by health plans to examine claims and determine benefits.

adjustment An amount (positive or negative) entered in a patient billing program to change a patient's account balance.

administrative simplification (AS) provisions of HIPAA Part of the federal law that requires a single national standard for each category of health care information, such as procedure codes.

admitting diagnosis The patient's condition determined by a physician at admission to an inpatient facility.

advance beneficiary notice (ABN) Medicare form used to inform a patient that a service to be provided is not likely to be reimbursed by the program.

aging report A report that shows the time span between issuing an invoice and receiving payment; used in medical offices to determine late payments and collect them.

allowed charge The maximum charge that a health plan pays for a specific service or procedure; also called allowable charge, maximum fee, and other terms.

Alphabetic Index The section of the ICD-9-CM in which diseases and injuries with corresponding diagnosis codes are presented in alphabetical order.

ambulatory care Outpatient care.

ambulatory patient classification (APC) A Medicare payment classification for outpatient services.

American Academy of Professional Coders (AAPC) National association that fosters the establishment and maintenance of professional, ethical, education, and certification standards for medical coding.

American Association of Medical Assistants National association that fosters the profession of medical assisting.

American Association for Medical Transcription   National association fostering the profession of medical transcription.

American Health Information Management Association (AHIMA)   National association of health information management professionals; promotes valid, accessible, yet confidential health information and advocates quality health care.

American Medical Association (AMA)   Member organization for physicians; goals are to promote the art and science of medicine, improve public health, and promote ethical, educational, and clinical standards for the medical profession.

American National Standards Institute (ANSI)   Organization that sets standards for electronic data interchange on a national level.

Accredited Standards Committee X12, Insurance Subcommittee (ASC X12N)   The ANSI-accredited standards development organization that maintains the administrative and financial electronic transactions standards adopted under HIPAA.

appeal   A request sent to a payer for reconsideration of a claim adjudication.

assignment of benefits   Authorization by policyholder that allows a health plan to pay benefits directly to a provider.

at-home recovery care   Assistance with the activities of daily living provided for a patient in the home.

attending physician   The clinician primarily responsible for the care of the patient from the beginning of a hospitalization.

audit   Methodical review; in medical insurance, a formal examination of a physician's accounting or patient medical records.

audit-edit claim response   Report from a receiver of an electronic claim transmitted to its sender regarding the status and completeness of the claim.

authorization   Document signed by a patient that permits release of particular medical information under the specific stated conditions.

B

balance billing   Collecting the difference between a provider's usual fee and a payer's lower allowed charge from the insured.

benefits   The amount of money a health plan pays for services covered in an insurance policy.

billing provider   The person or organization (often a clearinghouse or billing service) sending a HIPAA claim, as distinct from the pay-to provider that receives payment.

billing service   Company that provides billing and claims processing services.

birthday rule   The guideline that determines which of two parents with medical coverage has the primary insurance for a child; the parent whose day of birth is earlier in the calendar year is considered primary.

BlueCard Program   A Blue Cross and Blue Shield program that provides benefits for plan subscribers who are away from their local areas.

BlueCard Worldwide   The international component of the BlueCard Program that allows BCBS plan members traveling or living abroad to receive the benefits they would receive at home.

Blue Cross   A primarily nonprofit corporation that offers prepaid medical benefits for hospital services, and some outpatient, home care, and other institutional services.

Blue Cross and Blue Shield Association (BCBS)   The national licensing agency of Blue Cross and Blue Shield Plans.

Blue Shield   A primarily nonprofit corporation which offers prepaid medical benefits for physician, dental, and vision services, and other outpatient care.

bundled code   Single procedure code used to report a group of related procedures.

C

canines Two of the 32 permanent adult teeth.

CHAMPUS Now the TRICARE program; formerly the Civilian Health and Medical Program of the Uniformed Services (Army, Navy, Air Force, Marine Corps, Coast Guard, Public Health Service, and the National Oceanic and Atmospheric Administration) that serves spouses and children of active-duty service members, military retirees and their families, some former spouses, and survivors of deceased military members.

CHAMPVA The Civilian Health and Medical Program of the Veterans Administration (now known as the Department of Veterans Affairs) which shares health care costs for families of veterans with 100 percent service-connected disability and the surviving spouses and children of veterans who die from service-connected disabilities.

CHAMPVA for Life Program for beneficiaries who are both Medicare and CHAMPVA eligible; extends benefits to spouses or dependents who are age sixty-five and over.

CMS See Centers for Medicare and Medicaid Services.

CMS-1450 Paper claim for hospital services; also known as the UB-92.

CMS-1500 Paper claim for physician services.

CPT The abbreviation that refers to the American Medical Association's publication *Current Procedural Terminology.*

capitation Payment method in which a prepayment covers the provider's services to a plan member for a specified period of time.

capitation rate (cap rate) The contractually set periodic prepayment to a provider for specified services to each enrolled plan member.

carrier Health plan; also known as insurance company, payer, or third-party payer.

case Group of related data about a patient's personal/insurance account information and a particular medical condition.

cash flow The inflow of payments from patients and payers to a medical practice and the outflow from the practice of payments to suppliers and staff; based on the actual movement of money rather than amounts that are receivable or payable.

catastrophic cap The maximum annual amount a TRICARE beneficiary must pay for deductible and cost share.

category In the ICD-9-CM, a three-digit code used to classify a particular disease or injury.

Category II codes Optional CPT codes that track performance measures for a medical goal such as reducing tobacco use.

Category III codes Temporary codes for emerging technology, services, and procedures; to be used, rather than an unlisted code, when available.

categorically needy A person who receives assistance from government programs such as Temporary Assistance for Needy Families (TANF).

Centers for Medicare and Medicaid Services (CMS) Federal agency within the Department of Health and Human Services (HHS) that runs Medicare, Medicaid, Clinical Laboratories (under the CLIA program), and other governmental health programs.

certificate Term for Blue Cross and Blue Shield medical insurance policy.

charge master (or **charge ticket**) A hospital's list of the codes and charges for its services.

chief complaint (CC) A patient's description of the symptoms or other reasons for seeking medical care for a provider encounter.

chronic An illness or condition with a long duration.

Civilian Health and Medical Program of the Veterans Administration See CHAMPVA.

Civil Service Retirement System (CSRS) A disability program for employees of the federal government.

claim adjustment reason code Code used by a health plan on a remittance advice to describe payment information.

claim attachment Documentation that a provider sends to a payer in support of a health care claim.

claim control number Unique number assigned by the sender to a health care claim.

claim frequency code (claim reason submission code) A code reported on a HIPAA 837 claim that identifies the claim as original, replacement, or void/cancel action.

claim scrubber Software that checks claims to permit error correction for "clean" claims.

clean claim A claim that is accepted by a health plan for adjudication.

clearinghouse A company that converts, for a fee, nonstandard data formats into HIPAA standard transactions and transmits the data to health plans; or also handles the reverse process, changing HIPAA formatted transactions from health plans into nonstandard formats for providers.

code linkage The connection between a service and a patient's condition or illness; establishes the medical necessity of the procedure.

code set Alphabetic and/or numeric representations for data. Medical code sets are systems of medical terms that are required for HIPAA transactions. Administrative (nonmedical) code sets, such as taxonomy codes and Zip codes, are also used in HIPAA transactions.

coding The process of assigning numerical codes to diagnoses and procedures/services.

coexisting condition Additional illness that either has an effect on the patient's primary illness or is also treated during the encounter.

coinsurance The portion of charges that an insured person must pay for health care services after payment of the deductible amount; usually stated as a percentage.

compliance plan A medical practice's written plan for (a) the appointment of a compliance officer and committee, (b) a code of conduct for physicians' business arrangements and employees' compliance, (c) training plans, (d) properly prepared and updated coding tools such as job reference aids, encounter forms, and documentation templates, (e) rules for prompt identification and refunding of overpayments, and (f) ongoing monitoring and auditing of claim preparation.

consultation Service performed by a physician to advise a requesting physician about a patient's condition and care; the consultant does not assume responsibility for the patient's care and must send a written report back to the requestor.

conventions Typographic techniques or standard practices that provide visual guidelines for understanding printed material.

coordination of benefits (COB) A clause in an insurance policy that explains how the policy will pay if more than one insurance policy applies to the claim.

copayment An amount that a health plan requires a beneficiary to pay at the time of service for each health care encounter.

Correct Coding Initiative See **National Correct Coding Initiative.**

cost-share The term meaning coinsurance for a TRICARE or CHAMPVA beneficiary.

covered entity (CE) Under HIPAA, a health plan, clearinghouse, or provider that transmits any health information in electronic form in connection with a HIPAA transaction. In the law, "health plan" does not specifically include workers' compensation programs, property and casualty programs, or disability insurance programs.

crossover claim   Claim for services to a Medicare/ Medicaid beneficiary; Medicare is the primary payer and automatically transmits claim information to Medicaid as the secondary payer.

cross-reference   Directions in printed material that tell a reader where to look for additional information.

Current Dental Terminology (CDT-4)   Publication of the American Dental Association containing a standardized classification system for reporting dental procedures and services.

Current Procedural Terminology (CPT)   Publication of the American Medical Association containing the HIPAA-mandated standardized classification system for reporting medical procedures and services performed by physicians.

D

database   An organized collection of related data items having a specific structure.

data element   The smallest unit of information in a HIPAA transaction.

data format   An arrangement of electronic data for transmission.

day sheet   In a medical office, a report that summarizes the business day's charges and payments, drawn from all the patient ledgers for the day.

deductible   An amount that an insured person must pay, usually on an annual basis, for health care services before a health plan's payment begins.

Defense Enrollment Eligibility Reporting System (DEERS)   The worldwide database of TRICARE and CHAMPVA beneficiaries.

de-identified health information   Medical data from which individual identifiers have been removed; also known as a redacted or blinded record.

dentin   The hard material that fills 80 to 90 percent of the tooth.

Dentist's Pretreatment Estimate   A dentist's estimate of dental work required for a patient that is submitted to an insurance carrier before the service is performed.

Dentist's Statement of Actual Services   A dental claim form that reports the services a dentist has performed for a patient.

dependent   A person other than the insured, such as a spouse or child, who is covered under a health plan.

destination payer   In HIPAA claims, the health plan receiving the claim.

determination   A payer's decision regarding the benefits due for a claim.

diagnosis   A physician's opinion of the nature of a patient's illness or injury.

diagnosis code   The number assigned to a diagnosis in the *International Classification of Diseases.*

diagnosis-related groups (DRGs)   A system of analyzing conditions and treatments for similar groups of patients used to establish Medicare fees for hospital inpatient services.

direct payment   Payment for procedures that is made by an insurance company or a patient to a provider.

disability compensation program   A plan that reimburses the insured for lost income when the insured cannot work because of an illness or injury, whether or not it is work-related.

disallowed charge   An item on a remittance advice that identifies the difference between the allowable charge and the amount the physician charged for a service.

documentation   The systematic, logical, and consistent recording of a patient's health status—history, examinations, tests, results of treatments, and observations—in chronological order in a patient medical record.

downcode   A payer's review and reduction of a procedure code (often an E/M code) to a lower level than reported by the provider.

durable medical equipment (DME) Medicare term for reusable physical supplies such as wheelchairs and hospital beds that are ordered by the provider for use in the home; reported with HPCPS Level II codes.

Dx Abbreviation for diagnosis.

E

E code An alphanumeric ICD code for an external cause of injury or poisoning.

E/M code See evaluation and management codes.

Early and Periodic Screening, Diagnosis, and Treatment (EPSDT) Medicaid's prevention, early detection, and treatment program for eligible children under the age of 21.

edit In an electronic claim, a computer check for missing data or other mistakes, such as outdated codes.

electronic claim A health care claim that is transmitted electronically; also known as an electronic media claim (EMC).

electronic data interchange (EDI) The exchange (system to system) of data in a standardized format.

electronic funds transfer (EFT) Electronic routing of funds between banks.

electronic media Electronic storage media, such as hard drives and removable media, and transmission media used to exchange information already in electronic storage media, such as the Internet. Paper transmission via fax and voice transmission via telephone are not electronic transmission.

electronic remittance Payment made through electronic funds transfer.

electronic remittance advice See remittance advice.

emergency care Care received in a situation in which a delay in the treatment of the patient would lead to a significant increase in the threat to life or body part.

enamel The outer coating of the tooth.

encounter An office visit between a patient and a medical professional.

encounter form A listing of the diagnoses, procedures, and charges for a patient's visit; also called the superbill.

encryption A method of scrambling transmitted data so it cannot be deciphered without the use of a confidential process or key.

eponym A name or phrase that is formed from or based on a person's name; usually describes a condition or procedure associated with that person.

established patient A patient who has received professional services from a provider (or another provider with the same specialty in the same practice) within the past three years.

ethics Standards of conduct based on moral principles.

etiology The cause or origin of a disease.

etiquette Standards of professional behavior.

evaluation and management (E/M) codes Procedure codes that cover physicians' services performed to determine the optimum course for patient care; listed in the Evaluation and Management section of CPT.

excluded service A service specified in a medical insurance contract as not covered.

explanation of benefits (EOB) A document from a payer sent to a patient that shows how the amount of a benefit was determined.

explanation of Medicare benefits (EOMB) See Medicare Summary Notice.

F

family deductible A fixed, periodic amount that must be met by the combination of payments for covered services to each individual of an insured/dependent group before benefits from a payer begin.

Federal Employees' Compensation Act (FECA) A federal law that provides workers' compensation insurance for civilian employees of the federal government.

Federal Employee Health Benefits (FEHB) plan The health insurance plan that covers employees of the federal program.

Federal Employees Retirement System (FERS) Disability program for employees of the federal government.

Federal Insurance Contribution Act (FICA) The federal law that authorizes payroll deductions for the Social Security Disability Program.

Federal Medicaid Assistance Percentage (FMAP) Basis for federal government Medicaid allocations to individual states.

fee-for-service Method of charging under which a provider's payment is based on each service performed.

fee schedule List of charges for services performed.

final report A report filed by the physician in a state workers' compensation case when the patient is discharged.

first report of injury or illness A report filed in state workers' compensation cases that contains the employer's name and address, employee's supervisor, date and time of accident, geographic location of injury, and the patient's description of what happened.

fiscal agent An organization that processes claims for a government program.

fiscal intermediary A government contractor that processes claims for government programs; for Medicare, the fiscal intermediary (FI) processes Part A claims.

formulary A list of a health plan's selected drugs and their proper dosages; often a plan pays only for the drugs it lists.

fraud Intentional deceptive act to obtain a benefit.

G

gatekeeper See primary care physician.

gingivae (gingiva) The gums.

global period The number of days surrounding a surgical procedure during which all services relating to the procedure—preoperative, during the surgery, and postoperative—are considered part of the surgical package and are not additionally reimbursed.

group health plan Under HIPAA, an employee health plan that either has 50 or more participants or is administered by another business entity.

guardian An adult legally responsible for care and custody of a minor.

H

HCFA See Centers for Medicare and Medicaid Services.

HCFA-1450 See CMS-1450.

HCFA-1500 See CMS-1500.

health care claim An electronic transaction or a paper document filed with a health plan to receive benefits.

Health Care Financing Administration See Centers for Medicare and Medicaid Services.

Health Care Common Procedure Coding System (HCPCS) Procedure codes for Medicare claims, made up of CPT codes (Level I) and national codes (Level II).

health information management (HIM) Hospital department that organizes and maintains patient medical records; also profession devoted to managing, analyzing, and utilizing data vital for patient care, making it accessible to healthcare providers.

Health Insurance Portability and Accountability Act (HIPAA) of 1996 Federal act that set forth guidelines for standardizing the electronic data interchange of administrative and financial transactions, exposing fraud and abuse in government programs, and protecting the security and privacy of health information.

health maintenance organization (HMO) A managed health care system in which providers agree to offer health care to the organization's members for fixed periodic payments from the plan; usually members must receive medical services only from the plan's providers.

health plan Under HIPAA, an individual or group plan that either provides or pays for the cost of medical care, including group health plan, health insurance issuer, health maintenance organization, Medicare Part A or B, Medicaid, TRICARE, and other governmental and nongovernmental plans.

Health Savings Account An insurance plan under which an employer sets aside an annual amount an employee can use to pay for certain types of health care costs; also known as a medical savings account.

HIPAA claim Generic term for the HIPAA ASC X12N 837 professional health care claim transaction.

HIPAA Electronic Health Care Transactions and Code Sets (TCS) The HIPAA rule governing the electronic exchange of health information.

HIPAA National Identifier HIPPA-mandated identification systems for employers, health care providers, health plans, and patients; the NPI, National Provider System, and employer system are in place, health plan and patient systems are to be created.

HIPAA Privacy Rule Law that regulates the use and disclosure of patients' protected health information (PHI).

HIPAA Security Rule Law that requires covered entities to establish administrative, physical, and technical safeguards to protect the confidentiality, integrity, and availability of health information.

HIPAA transaction General term for the electronic transactions, such as claim status inquiries, health care claim transmittal, and coordination of benefits regulated under the HIPAA Health Care Transactions and Code Sets standards.

home plan A Blue Cross and Blue Shield plan in the community where the subscriber has contracted for coverage.

hospice A public or private organization that provides services for terminally ill people and their families.

host plan A participating provider's local Blue Cross and Blue Shield plan.

I

ICD-9-CM Abbreviated title of *International Classification of Diseases, 9th Revision, Clinical Modification.*

ICD code A system of diagnostic codes based on the *International Classification of Diseases.*

incisors Four of the 32 permanent adult teeth; the cutting teeth.

indemnity plan An insurance company's agreement to reimburse a policyholder a predetermined amount for covered losses.

indirect payment Payment made to a provider by an insurance company on behalf of a patient.

individual deductible A fixed, periodic amount that must be met by each individual of an insured/dependent group before benefits from a payer begin.

informed consent The process by which a patient authorizes medical treatment after discussion regarding the nature, indications, benefits, and risks of a treatment a physician recommends.

inpatient A person admitted to a medical facility for services that require an overnight stay.

insurance aging report A report grouping unpaid claims transmitted to payers by the length of time that they remain due, such as 30, 60, 90, or 120 days.

insurance carrier Health plan; also known as insurance company, payer, or third-party payer.

insured The policyholder or subscriber to a health plan or medical insurance policy; also known as guarantor.

***International Classification of Diseases, 9th Revision, Clinical Modification* (ICD-9-CM)** A publication containing the HIPAA-mandated standardized classification system for diseases and injuries; developed by the World Health Organization and modified for use in the United States.

L

liable Legally responsible.

limiting charge In Medicare, the highest fee (115 percent of the Medicare Fee Schedule) that nonparticipating physicians can charge for a particular service.

line item control number On a HIPAA claim, the unique number assigned by the sender to each service line item reported.

M

main number The five-digit procedure code listed in the CPT.

main term The word in bold-faced type that identifies a disease or condition in the Alphabetic index in ICD-9-CM.

managed care A system that combines the financing and the delivery of appropriate, cost-effective health care services to its members.

managed care organization (MCO) Organization offering some type of managed health care plan.

mandible The lower jaw bone.

master patient index A hospital's main patient database.

maxilla The upper jaw bone.

maxillofacial surgery Surgical procedure related to the face and jaw.

Medicaid A federal and state assistance program that pays for health care services for people who cannot afford them.

MediCal California's state Medicaid program name.

medical insurance A financial plan that covers the cost of hospital and medical care due to illness or injury.

medical insurance specialist The person in a medical office who handles patients' health care claims.

medical malpractice Failure to use an acceptable level of professional skill when giving medical services that results in injury or harm to a patient.

medical necessity Payment criterion of payers that requires medical treatments to be appropriate and provided in accordance with generally accepted standards of medical practice. The reported procedure or service (1) matches the diagnosis, (2) is not elective, (3) is not experimental, (4) has not been performed for the convenience of the patient or the patient's family, and (5) has been provided at the appropriate level.

medical necessity denial Refusal by a health plan to pay for a reported procedure that does not meet its medical necessity criteria.

medical record A file that contains the documentation of a patient's medical history, record of care, progress notes, correspondence, and related billing/financial information.

medically indigent Medically needy.

medically needy Medicaid classification for people with high medical expenses and low financial resources, although not sufficiently low to receive cash assistance.

Medicare The federal health insurance program for people 65 or older and some people with disabilities.

Medicare Advantage Medicare plans other than the Original Medicare Plan.

Medicare beneficiary A person covered by Medicare.

Medicare carrier A private organization under contract with CMS to administer Medicare Part B claims in an assigned region.

Medicare Fee Schedule (MFS) The RBRVS-based allowed fees that are reimbursable to Medicare participating physicians.

Medicare Modernization Act (MMA) Short name for the Medicare Prescription Drug, Improvement, and Modernization Act of 2003, which includes a number of changes that will roll out over a period of years, including a prescription drug benefit.

Medicare Part A The part of the Medicare program that pays for hospitalization, care in a skilled nursing facility, home health care, and hospice care.

Medicare Part B The part of the Medicare program that pays for physician services, outpatient hospital services, durable medical equipment, and other services and supplies.

Medicare-participating agreement A phrase that describes physicians and other providers of medical services who have signed agreements with Medicare to accept assignment on all Medicare claims.

Medicare Remittance Notice (MRN) Remittance advice from Medicare to providers that explains how payments for a batch of Medicare claims were determined.

Medicare Summary Notice (MSN) Type of remittance advice from Medicare to plan beneficiaries to explain how their benefits were determined.

Medigap Insurance plan offered by a private insurance carrier to supplement Medicare Original Plan coverage.

Medi-Medi beneficiary Person who is eligible for both Medicare and Medicaid benefits.

member plan Independent insurance company licensed to offer Blue Cross and Blue Shield health plans.

military treatment facility (MTF) Government facility providing medical services for members and dependents of the Uniformed Services.

minimum necessary standard Principle that individually identifiable health information should be disclosed only to the extent needed to support the purpose of the disclosure.

modifier A number that is appended to a code to report particular facts. CPT modifiers report special circumstances involved with a procedure or service. HCPCS modifiers are often used to designate a body part, such as left side or right side.

molars Six of the 32 permanent adult teeth.

N

National Correct Coding Initiative (NCCI) Computerized Medicare system to prevent overpayment for procedures.

National Patient ID (Individual Identifier) Unique individual identification system to be created under HIPAA National Identifiers.

National Payer ID (Health Plan ID) Unique health plan identification system to be created under HIPAA National Identifiers.

National Provider Identifier (NPI) Under HIPAA, unique 10-digit identifier assigned to each provider by the National Provider System; replaces both the UPIN and Medicare PIN.

National Uniform Claim Committee (NUCC) Organization responsible for the content of health care claims.

nationwide plan A Blue Cross and Blue Shield national account health plan.

network model HMO A type of health maintenance organization where physicians remain self-employed and provide services to both HMO-members and nonmembers.

new patient A patient who has not received professional services from a provider (or another provider with the same specialty in the same practice) within the past three years.

nonavailability statement (NAS) A form required for preauthorization when a TRICARE member seeks medical services in other than military treatment facilities.

nonparticipating (nonPAR) physician A physician or other health care provider who chooses not to join a particular government or other program or plan.

nontraumatic injury   A condition caused by the work environment over a period longer than one work day or shift. Also known as occupational disease or illness.

not elsewhere classified (NEC)   An ICD-9-CM abbreviation indicating the code to be used when an illness or condition cannot be placed in any other category.

Notice of Claim Filed   Notification from Social Security that a patient of a medical office has filed for disability compensation.

Notice of Exclusions from Medicare Benefits (NEMB)   CMS form that can be used by participating providers to give Medicare patients, before providing an uncovered service such as a screening test, written notification that Medicare will not pay and the estimated charge for which the patient will be responsible.

Notice of Privacy Practices (NPP)   A HIPAA-mandated description of a covered entity's principles and procedures related to the protection of patients' health information.

not otherwise specified (NOS)   An ICD-9-CM abbreviation indicating the code to be used when no information is available for assigning the illness or condition a more specific code.

O

occlusion   The contact between the upper and lower teeth.

occupational disease/illness   A condition caused by the work environment over a period longer than one work day or shift; also known as nontraumatic injury.

Occupational Safety and Health Administration (OSHA)   Federal agency that regulates workers' health and safety risks in the workplace.

Office of Civil Rights (OCR)   Government agency that enforces the HIPAA Privacy Act.

Office of the Inspector General (OIG)   Government agency that investigates and prosecutes fraud against government health care programs such as Medicare.

Office of Workers' Compensation Programs (OWCP)   The office of the U.S. Department of Labor that administers the Federal Employees' Compensation Act.

OIG Compliance Program Guidance for Individual and Small Group Physician Practices   OIG publication that explains the recommended features of compliance plans for small providers.

oral cavity   The inner section of the mouth.

oral surgery   Surgical procedure related to the face and jaw.

Original Medicare Plan   The Medicare fee-for-service plan.

out-of-area program   A Blue Cross and Blue Shield Association program that provides benefits for subscribers who are away from their local areas.

out-of-pocket   Expenses the insured must pay before benefits begin.

outpatient   A patient who receives health care in a hospital setting without admission; the length of stay is generally less than 23 hours.

overpayment   An improper or excessive payment to a provider as a result of billing or claims processing errors for which a refund is owed by the provider.

P

palate   The roof of the mouth.

panel   In CPT, a single code grouping laboratory tests that are frequently done together.

participating (PAR) physician/provider   A physician/provider who agrees to provide medical services to a payer's policyholders according to the terms of the plan or program's contract.

password   Confidential authentication information composed of a string of characters.

patient aging report   A report grouping unpaid patients' bills by the length of time that they remain due, such as 30, 60, 90, or 120 days.

patient information form A form that includes a patient's personal, employment, and insurance company data needed to complete a health care claim; also known as a registration form.

patient ledger A record of all charges and payments made on a particular patient's account.

patient statement A report that shows the services provided to a patient, the total payments made, total charges, adjustments, and the balance due.

payer Insurance carrier; also known as insurance company, health plan, or third-party payer.

payer of last resort Regulation that Medicaid pays last on a claim when a patient has other insurance coverage.

pay-to provider The person or organization that is to receive payment for services reported on a HIPAA claim; may be the same as or different from the billing provider.

permanent disability A condition that prevents a person with a disability compensation program from doing any job.

place of service (POS) code A HIPAA administrative code that indicates where medical services have been provided, such as an office or hospital.

point-of-service (POS) plan In HMOs, a plan that permits patients to receive medical services from non-network providers; this choice requires a larger patient payment than visits with network providers.

policyholder A person who buys an insurance plan; the insured, subscriber, or guarantor.

preauthorization Prior authorization from a payer for services to be provided; if not received, the charge is not usually covered.

preexisting condition An illness or disorder of a beneficiary that existed before the effective date of insurance coverage.

preferred provider organization (PPO) A managed care organization structured as a network of health care providers who agree to perform services for plan members at discounted fees; usually, plan members can receive services from non-network providers for a higher charge.

premium The periodic amount of money the insured pays to a health plan for a health care policy.

premolars Four of the 32 permanent adult teeth.

preventive medical services Care that is provided to keep patients healthy or to prevent illness, such as routine checkups and screening tests.

Primary Care Manager (PCM) Provider who coordinates and manages the care of TRICARE beneficiaries.

primary care physician (PCP) A physician in a health maintenance organization who directs all aspects of a patient's care, including routine services, referrals to specialists within the system, and supervision of hospital admissions; also known as a gatekeeper.

primary diagnosis A diagnosis that represents the patient's major illness or condition for an encounter.

primary insurance (payer) The health plan that pays benefits first when a patient is covered by more than one plan.

primary procedure The most resource-intensive (highest paid) CPT procedure done during a patient's encounter.

principal diagnosis The condition that after study is established as chiefly responsible for a patient's admission to a hospital.

principal procedure The main service performed for the condition listed as the principal diagnosis for a hospital inpatient.

prior authorization number An identifying code assigned by a government program or health insurance plan when preauthorization is required; also called the certification number.

private disability insurance   An insurance plan that can be purchased to provide the insured benefits when illness or injury prevents employment.

procedure code   A code that identifies medical treatment or diagnostic services.

prognosis   The physician's prediction of outcome of disease and likelihood of recovery.

progress report   A report filed by the physician in state workers' compensation cases when a patient's medical condition or disability changes; also known as a supplemental report.

prophylaxes   Dental procedure to clean the teeth.

Prospective Payment System (PPS)   Medicare system for payment for institutional services.

prostheses   Dental bridges and dentures.

protected health information (PHI)   Individually identifiable health information that is transmitted or maintained by electronic media.

provider   A person or entity that supplies medical or health services and bills for or is paid for the services in the normal course of business. A provider may be a professional member of the health care team, such as a physician, or a facility, such as a hospital or skilled nursing home.

pulp   The soft core of the tooth containing the nerves and blood vessels.

R

reasonable fee   The lower of either the fee the physician bills or the usual fee, unless special circumstances apply.

referral   Transfer of patient care from one physician to another.

referral number   Authorization number given by a referring physician to the referred physician.

referring provider   The physician who refers the patient to another physician for treatment.

registration   The process of gathering personal and insurance information about a patient during admission to a hospital.

relative value scale (RVS)   System of assigning unit values to medical services based on an analysis of the skill and time required of the physician to perform them.

relative value unit (RVU)   A factor assigned to a medical service based on the relative skill and time required to perform it.

remittance   The statement of the results of the health plan's adjudication of a claim.

remittance advice (RA)   Health plan document describing a payment resulting from a claim adjudication; also called an explanation of benefits (EOB).

rendering provider   Term used to identify the physician or other medical professional who provides the procedure reported on a health care claim if other than the pay-to provider.

Resource-Based Relative Value Scale (RBRVS)   Federally mandated relative value scale for establishing Medicare charges.

responsible party   Person or entity other than the insured or the patient who will pay a patient's charges.

retention schedule   A practice policy that governs which information from patients' medical records is to be stored, for how long it is to be retained, and the storage medium to be used.

rider   Document that modifies an insurance contract.

S

schedule of benefits   A list of the medical expenses that a health plan covers.

secondary insurance (payer)   The health plan that pays benefits after the primary plan when a patient is covered by more than one plan.

secondary procedure   A procedure performed in addition to the primary procedure.

secondary provider identifier   On HIPAA claims, identifiers that may be required by various plans in addition to the NPI, such as a plan identification number.

self-insured employer   A company that creates its own insurance plan for its employees, rather than using a carrier; the employer assumes all payment risk, contracts with physicians, and pays for claims from a company fund.

self-pay patient   A patient who does not have insurance coverage.

service line information   On a HIPAA claim, information about the services being reported.

small health plan   Under HIPAA, a health plan with under $5 million in annual receivables.

Social Security Disability Insurance (SSDI)   The federal disability compensation program for salaried and hourly wage earners, self-employed people who pay a special tax, and widows, widowers, and minor children with disabilities whose deceased spouse/parent would qualify for Social Security benefits if alive.

sponsor   The uniformed service member in a family qualified for TRICARE or CHAMPVA.

staff model HMO   A type of HMO in which member providers are employees of the organization and provide services only for HMO-member patients.

State Children's Health Insurance Program (SCHIP)   Program to offer health insurance coverage for uninsured children under Medicaid.

state compensation board/commission   The state agency that administers state workers' compensation laws.

State Disability Insurance (SDI)   State-based disability insurance program that covers all the employees in a state.

subcategory   In ICD-9-CM, a four-digit code number.

subclassification   In ICD-9-CM, a five-digit code number.

subpoena   A order of a court for a party to appear and testify in a court of law.

subpoena *duces tecum*   An order of a court directing a party to appear, to testify, and to bring specified documents or items.

subscriber   The insured.

subterm   A word or phrase that describes a main term in the Alphabetic Index of the ICD-9-CM.

superbill   A listing of the diagnoses, procedures, and charges for a patient's visit; also called the encounter form.

supplemental insurance   An insurance plan, such as Medigap, that provides benefits for services which are not normally covered by a primary plan.

supplemental report   A report filed by the physician in state workers' compensation cases when a patient's medical condition or disability changes; also known as progress report.

Supplemental Security Income (SSI)   A government program that helps pay living expenses for low-income older people and those who are blind or have disabilities.

supplementary term   A nonessential word or phrase that helps to define a code in the ICD-9-CM; usually enclosed in parentheses or brackets.

surgical package   A combination of services included in a single procedure code for some surgical procedures in CPT.

T

Tabular List   The section of the ICD-9-CM in which diagnosis codes are presented in numerical order.

taxonomy code   Administrative code set under HIPAA that is used to report a physician's specialty when it affects payment.

Temporary Assistance for Needy Families (TANF)   A government program that provides cash assistance for low-income families.

temporary disability   A condition that keeps a person with a private disability compensation program from working at the usual job for a short time, but from which the worker is expected to recover completely and return to work.

third-party liability   An obligation of an insurance plan or government program to pay all or part of medical costs.

third-party payer   A private or governmental organization that insures or pays for health care on the behalf of beneficiaries: The insured person is the first party, the provider the second party, and the payer the third party.

trace number   A number assigned to a HIPAA 270 electronic transaction sent to a health plan to inquire about patient eligibility for benefits.

transaction   Under HIPAA, a structured set of data transmitted between two parties to carry out financial or administrative activities related to health care; in a medical billing program, a financial exchange that is recorded, such as a patient's copayment or deposit of funds into the provider's bank account.

traumatic injury   An injury caused by a specific event or series of events within a single work day or shift.

treatment, payment, and operations (TPO)   Health care treatment, payment, and operations; under HIPAA, patients' protected health information may be shared for TPO.

TRICARE   A government health program that serves dependents of active-duty service members, military retirees and their families, some former spouses, and survivors of deceased military members; formerly called CHAMPUS.

TRICARE Extra   TRICARE'S managed care health plan that offers a network of civilian providers.

TRICARE for Life   Program for beneficiaries who are both Medicare and TRICARE eligible.

TRICARE Prime   The basic managed care health plan offered by TRICARE.

TRICARE Standard   The fee-for-service health plan offered by TRICARE.

U

UB-92   Paper hospital claim, formerly a Medicare-required Part A (hospital) form; also known as the CMS-1450.

unbundling   The incorrect billing practice of breaking a panel or package of services/procedures into component parts and reporting them separately.

uncollectible accounts   Monies that cannot be collected from the practice's payers or patients and must be written off.

unlisted procedure   A service that is not listed in CPT; reported with an unlisted procedure code and requires a special report when used.

upcode   Use of a procedure code that provides a higher payment than the code for the service actually provided.

urgently needed care   In Medicare, a beneficiary's unexpected illness or injury requiring immediate treatment; Medicare plans pay for this service even if it is provided outside of a plan's service area.

usual, customary, and reasonable (UCR)   Setting fees by comparing the usual fee the provider charges for the service, the customary fee charged by most providers in the community, and what is reasonable considering the circumstances.

usual fee   Fee for a service or procedure that is charged by a provider for most patients under typical circumstances.

uvula   The cone-shaped structure at the end of the soft palate.

V

V code   An alphanumeric code in the ICD-9-CM that identifies factors that influence health status and encounters that are not due to illness or injury.

verification report   A report created by a medical billing program to permit double-checking of basic claim content before transmission.

Veteran's Compensation Program   A federal disability program covering veterans of the uniformed services.

Veteran's Pension Program   A federal disability program covering veterans of the uniformed services.

W

walkout receipt   A medical billing program report given to a patient that lists the diagnoses, services provided, fees, and payments received and due after an encounter.

Welfare Reform Act   1996 law that established the Temporary Assistance for Needy Families program in place of the Aid to Families with Dependent Children program and tightened Medicaid eligibility requirements.

workers' compensation insurance   A state or federal plan that covers medical care and other benefits for employees who suffer accidental injury or become ill as a result of employment.

write off   (N. write-off) To deduct an amount from a patient's account because of a contractual agreement to accept a payer's allowed charge or other reason.

Index